ABC OF SEXUAL HEALTH

Second Edition

ABC OF SEXUAL HEALTH

Second Edition

Edited by

JOHN M TOMLINSON

Specialist in sexual health, Royal Hampshire County Hospital, Winchester
Formerly general practitioner and honorary senior lecturer in primary care,
University of Southampton

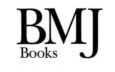

BMJ
Books

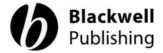

Blackwell
Publishing

Blackwell Publishing, Inc., 350 Main Street, Malden, Massachusetts 02148-5020, USA
Blackwell Publishing Ltd, 9600 Garsington Road, Oxford OX4 2DQ, UK
Blackwell Publishing Asia Pty Ltd, 550 Swanston Street, Carlton, Victoria 3053, Australia

First published 1999
Second edition 2005

Library of Congress Cataloging-in-Publication Data
ABC of sexual health / edited by John M. Tomlinson—2nd ed.
        p. ;   cm.
   Includes bibliographical references and index.
   ISBN 0-7279-1759-5
   1. Sexual disorders. 2.   Psychosexual disorders.
   [DNLM: 1. Sex Disorders. 2.   Sexual Behavior.   WP 610 A134 2004]   I.   Tomlinson, John M., physician.

RC556.A23 2004
616.6′9—dc22

2004014019

ISBN 0 7279 1759 5

A catalogue record for this title is available from the British Library

Cover image is of *Formality of Couples* 1998 by Emily Young with permission

Set in 9/11 pt by Newgen Imaging Systems (P) Ltd, Chennai, India
Printed and bound in India by Replika Press Pvt. Ltd

Commissioning Editor: Eleanor Lines
Development Editors: Sally Carter/Nick Morgan
Production Controller: Kate Charman

For further information on Blackwell Publishing, visit our website:
http://www.blackwellpublishing.com

The publisher's policy is to use permanent paper from mills that operate a sustainable forestry policy, and which has been manufactured from pulp processed using acid-free and elementary chlorine-free practices. Furthermore, the publisher ensures that the text paper and cover board used have met acceptable environmental accreditation standards.

Contents

Contributors

Robin Bell
Formerly genitourinary medicine practitioner, St Mary's Hospital, London

Josie Butcher
General practitioner, Nantwich; director of the Psychosexual Counselling Service, Cheshire and Wirral Partnership Trust; and leader in psychosexual therapy MSc course, University of Central Lancashire

John Dean
Locum consultant in sexual medicine, Devon Partnership NHS Trust

Christine Evans
Consultant urologist, North Wales

Clive Glass
Consultant clinical psychologist, regional spinal injuries unit, Southport District General Hospital

Alain Gregoire
Consultant psychiatrist, Hampshire Partnership Trust, Tatchbury Mount Hospital, Southampton

Ruth Hallam-Jones
Sexual psychotherapist and senior nurse, Porterbrook clinic, Royal Hallamshire Hospital, Sheffield

Christopher Headon
Psychosexual therapist, Albany Trust, London

Margot Huish
Sex and relationship therapist, Barnet, Enfield and Haringay Mental Health NHS Trust, Barnet Hospital

Roger S Kirby
Professor of urology, St George's Hospital, London

Asun de Marquiegui
Sex therapist and instructing doctor in family planning, King's College Hospital, London

Tony Parsons
Consultant gynaecologist, University Hospitals of Coventry and Warwickshire NHS Trust and senior lecturer, Warwick Medical School

Margaret Ramage
Tutor in human sexuality, St George's Hospital, London

Jane Read
Sex relationship therapist London, and Edinburgh

Margaret Rees
Reader in reproductive medicine, University of Oxford and consultant in medical gynaecology, John Radcliffe Hospital, Oxford

Padmal de Silva
Consultant clinical psychologist, Maudsley Hospital, London and senior lecturer in clinical psychology

Bakulesh Soni
Consultant in spinal injuries, regional spinal injuries unit, Southport District General Hospital

John M Tomlinson
Specialist in sexual health, Royal Hampshire County Hospital, Winchester; formerly general practitioner and honorary senior lecturer in primary care, University of Southampton

Kevan Wylie
Consultant in sexual medicine, Porterbrook Clinic and consultant andrologist, Royal Hallamshire Hospital, Sheffield

Foreword

Individuals, the press, and society often find it difficult to handle and deal with sexual matters and sexual identity. The medical profession, as members of the public, will at times grapple with their own sexual orientation and problems, and have varying views and value systems around sexual matters and morality, and of course why not? They have a responsibility, however, to be well informed about sexual health so that they can educate and help patients at the same time as adopting a neutral and non-censorious position. It is bad manners and bad medicine to force one's own personal moral attitudes and beliefs about sexual matters on patients.

Sexual health is badly covered in the undergraduate curriculum, so doctors are not as knowledgeable and comfortable about this area of medicine to be of most help to their patients. In light of this, the *ABC of Sexual Health* is to be warmly welcomed. This second edition of the *ABC of Sexual Health* is a much more detailed examination of sexual problems and variations. This only makes sense if done in an open and explicit fashion, and covers a wide variety of sexual habits and practices. Ultimately, this approach will help us to understand a range of problems and behaviours so as to be able to deal with everyday issues presented by our patients. This book will put the profession in touch with the real world, real people with real problems, and fill a large gap in our knowledge.

Michael W Adler
Professor of Sexually Transmitted Diseases
Department of Sexually Transmitted Diseases
Royal Free and University College Medical School
London

Preface

Preface to the second edition

This ABC is intended to be an update and a summary of a wide range of sexual matters and will, I hope, be a help to those who want to be more informed about the subject. It is not intended to be totally inclusive and some subjects could not be covered fully, so there are many references for further reading. There are two new chapters—on transsexualism and transvestism, and the latest information up to the time of publication on current views of hormone replacement therapy in females and males.

I am grateful for those who have made helpful comments and suggestions after publication of the series when it came out in the *BMJ* and later as a book, and I hope that all corrections have been made.

From the preface to the first edition

When I was a course organiser for general practitioner registrars, they made frequent requests for help with psychosexual problems that they came across in the course of their work, as none of them had had any training in human sexuality.[1] Unfortunately, with some notable exceptions, this still seems to be the case.

Although there are many sources of information on sex, presented with great openness and frankness, they are not necessarily accurate and there has been a lack of authoritative information on sexuality and all its variations for those practitioners who might come across sexual problems incidental to their professional work, and for medical and nursing students. This collection of articles has attempted to fill such a gap.

I hope that the *ABC of Sexual Health* will make a contribution to informing and helping doctors, other health professionals and students (of all professions) to talk about sexual matters with more ease.

1 Weston JAB, Tomlinson JM. The Guildford (University of Surrey) release course for trainee practitioners. *J R Coll Gen Pract* 1984;**34**:82-6.

Acknowledgements

My thanks are due to Richard Smith, former editor of the *BMJ*, who encouraged the Editorial Board to publish this series in the journal, as well as to Greg Cotton, technical editor, Jan Croot, pictures editor, Sally Carter, development editor, and Eleanor Lines, ABC series commissioning editor, for their patience and help at all times. I am also grateful to Daryl Higgins and Simon Vearnals who both gave many constructive ideas and much help with the new edition.

John M Tomlinson

1 Management of sexual problems

Margaret Ramage

Sexual problems present in various ways, often indirectly or covertly. Patients do not like to come straight to the point. They fear looking stupid by using wrong words or giving offence by being too explicit, or they have no way of conceptualising what is wrong. Doctors can find themselves fumbling around in a slightly mad conversation in which nobody understands what is being said. A common language needs to be established first, particularly in sexual medicine, followed by a good history and careful examination, if appropriate, before an assessment of relevant management can be made. Recurrent gynaecological or urological complaints, insomnia, depression, joint pains, and other symptoms have all been used as covert presentations of sexual problems.

Once the presence of a sexual problem has been established, the severity and importance to the patient need to be determined so that the most appropriate course of management can be offered. This can vary from straightforward education—simply giving accurate information—to referral for psychiatric assessment (happily very rare). History taking therefore is the paramount skill that underpins decisions about management, but formation of a positive alliance with the patient also is vital. Any course of action has to have complete cooperation: without that, the best treatment in the world may be useless.

Overall management

Worth bearing in mind is that however obviously physical the cause of a sexual problem, psychological sequelae may well be present—if not for the patient then for his or her partner if there is one. Conversely, when the cause seems to be entirely psychological, hidden organic factors may exist, and it would be irresponsible to miss them. Overall management therefore has to take account of both aspects (exclusion of organic factors is covered in Chapter 5).

Psychological approaches

The sexual arousal circuit

A challenge for clinicians is to enable patients to understand that sexual problems happen in response to something and usually are not located solely in the genitals. Relationships, early learning about sex, trauma, and life stresses all can contribute. The sexual arousal circuit can be used to show how these factors all may be linked to the sexual problem and to explain that sexual arousal at its simplest may be a straightforward spinal reflex triggered by stimulation of the genital area.[1] This is interpreted in the brain and moderated by the emotions, so that events in the two arenas will exert a powerful influence over that reflex. Sexual response can be described as an electrical circuit that can start anywhere—in the mind, the body, or the emotions—but that also has three breakpoints: one in each area.

The *first breakpoint* occurs when inappropriate stimulation or pain occurs. For many people, pain can automatically cancel any possibility of response. Common problems are inappropriate stimulation of the clitoris and in particular insufficient stimulation of the penis in older men—a point not appreciated widely.

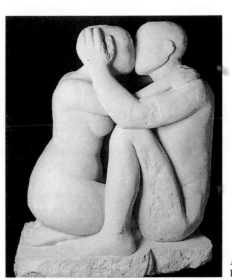

Man, woman and fish by Emily Young

Useful guides

Videos and DVDs
- *Sex, a lifelong pleasure* (a series of three videos). Great Dunmow: Press Play (tel: 01371 873138)
- *Lovers' guide* (a series introduced by Dr Andrew Stanway). London: Carlton Home Entertainment (tel: 020 8207 6207)

Both of these videos are 10 years old, but the information in the first of each scene is helpful

Books
- Zilbergeld B. *The new male sexuality.* London: Bantam, 1999
- Quilliam S. *A woman's complete illustrated guide to sex.* London: Fair Winds Press, 2003
- Litvinoff S. *Relate: sex in loving relationships.* London: Vermilion, 2001

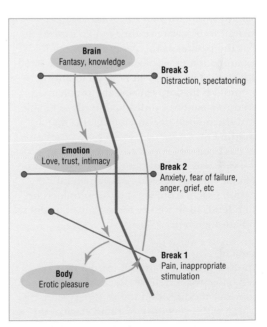

The sexual arousal circuit, a schematic representation of the factors that can positively or negatively affect the sexual response in the body, the mind, and the emotions

The *second breakpoint* occurs when the mind is too busy for the person to relax and become aroused. An example of this, common in men with erectile or ejaculatory dysfunction, is "spectatoring," when the mind is focused on observing the performance of the penis to the exclusion of almost everything else. Other examples include distraction caused by worries about work, memories of negative experiences, expectations of failure, uncertainty of how to behave, and many others.

The third breakpoint (and probably the most powerful) occurs in the emotional arena, and a patient can be paralysed by fear of failure, anxiety, and pressure to perform. Other negative emotions important in this context include anger, unresolved conflict (in any area of life), undisclosed resentment, and grief.

Giving accurate information
Accurate information can be all that is needed to resolve some sexual problems: for example, when patients lack knowledge of the basics of sexual anatomy and physiology, the changes of ageing or have unrealistic ideas of what is "normal." It can be particularly invaluable to women who have never examined themselves or men worried about the size of their genitals.

General counselling
Counselling can uncover and help resolve hidden conflicts or long denied emotions of anger and grief. Any relationship issues may be explored in this context, and communication between partners, which often is difficult in the presence of sexual problems, can be facilitated. Realistic goals can be established, and lifestyle changes (diet, exercise, and general fitness) can be agreed and supported. An environment of emotional support and understanding can help patients work out their own solutions.

Psychosexual therapy
The assumption that underlies psychosexual therapy is that the relationship between therapist and patient provides a mirror of the relationship between the patient and his or her partner. It enables understanding of any disturbed interaction with the partner and hidden conflicts in the patient. Initially, the doctor asks questions only when necessary to minimise leading the patient. Medical investigations and questioning sometimes can be a way of avoiding painful and important emotional matters that the patient or doctor may be afraid to face.

It is most important to be aware of the feelings evoked in the doctor as well as the patient as the patient's story unfolds and the physical examination takes place. These feelings need to be discussed with the patient and can be used to inform them of the inner conflicts that are causing the problems. Treatment is tailored to a patient's individual needs to enable an understanding of the unique unconscious blocks that are hindering sexual fulfilment.

This technique has been developed to be useful in a relatively short interview and so does not necessarily need any commitment to regular therapy sessions. Many general practitioners and some practice nurses have been trained in this approach, which lends itself well to the setting of a general practice or family planning clinic.

Behavioural approach
Patients with compulsive sexual behaviour, including paraphilia, are likely to be treated most effectively with a programme of behaviour modification under supervision (see Chapter 11). Men with premature or rapid ejaculation can learn to delay ejaculation through a programme of graded masturbatory exercises (the squeeze technique), with or without drug treatment. These exercises aim to enable a patient

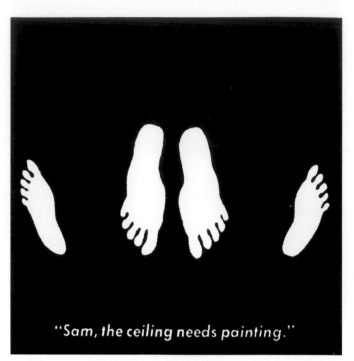

"Sam, the ceiling needs painting."

The second break point in the sexual arousal circuit occurs when the mind is too busy for the person to relax and become aroused

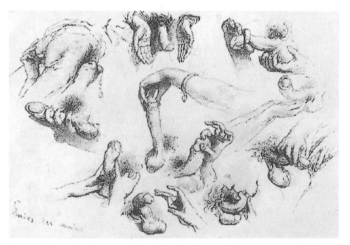

Counselling can uncover and help resolve hidden conflicts or long denied anger and grief

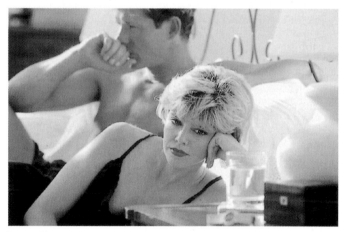

By modifying the stimulation in masturbatory exercises, a man with premature ejaculation can learn to slow his response. (Studies of masturbation from *Love* (1911) by Mihaly von Zichy)

to recognise the feelings in his penis at different levels of arousal and to slow the response by modifying the stimulation. Vaginismus also can be dealt with through behavioural approaches (see Chapter 7).

Sexual and relationship therapy

This integrated therapy incorporates psychodynamic, behavioural, cognitive, and systemic principles. The relationship may be viewed as "the patient" rather the partners being viewed as individuals. After thorough assessment of physical, psychological, and relationship factors, particularly if a couple attends sessions together, a therapeutic contract is made, with clearly stated goals, if possible, and sometimes a limited number of sessions. The patient or couple may agree to "homework" to facilitate and maintain changes. Family influences and cultural and gender issues also may be important, and communication between partners often is fundamental in this approach. With a sexual problem, the relationship inevitably will be affected, but this commonly can offer the vehicle to ameliorate the situation.

Once communication between partners is open and constructive, therapeutic tasks can be assigned to enable them to resolve their difficulties in the privacy of their own home and at times to suit their lifestyle. The therapist's job is to work out with the couple what would be most helpful. The feedback from these tasks, together with the appropriate management of any important emotional material that arises from them, provides the route by which many sexual problems can be resolved.

Sensate focus

Sensate focus is a programme of tasks that a couple can undertake in their own time at home. First described by Masters and Johnson in 1970,[2] it has been evolving and developing ever since.[3] A ban on sexual intercourse and any genital contact underlies the programme until performance anxiety and fear of failure have subsided and trust between the couple is established. This ban ensures that physical intimacy will not lead to sexual intimacy. The tasks involve the couple setting aside time to explore each other's bodies in turn by touching, stroking, caressing, and massaging. Sensual, then erotic, and then sexual touch are introduced gradually over time.

Ground rules need to be acceded to, the couple's progress monitored, and the next set of tasks agreed, to deal with any issues that may arise as a result of the tasks, support positive changes, and prevent relapse in the early stages. Suggested ground rules are:

- Agree a ban on sexual intercourse and genital touching
- Set up twice weekly times to spend on this homework, increasing from 20 minutes to 60 minutes over four weeks
- During these times, speak only if the partner's touch is painful or unacceptable; otherwise what is being done is assumed to be acceptable. Conversation will prevent concentration on the task and render it pointless
- Attention should focus on personal experience, not on pleasing the partner
- Above all, this is a learning exercise.

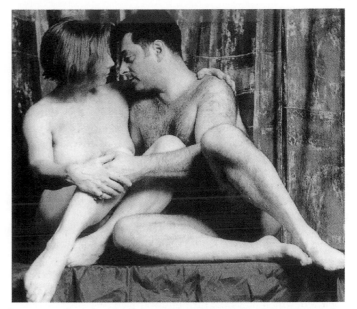

Partners can be assigned tasks to enable them to resolve their difficulties in the privacy of their own home

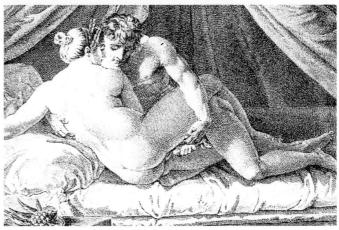

In sensate focus, the couple explore each other's bodies by touching, stroking and caressing. (*Antoine et Cleopatre* (circa 1602) by Agostino Carracci)

Sensate focus

Stage 1

1—Each person takes plenty of time to explore each other's naked (if possible) body, avoiding the breasts and genitals, avoiding trying to give pleasure, and concentrating on feelings and sensations experienced in both "active" and "passive" roles

2—After two weeks or four sessions of this, some familiarity and trust should allow inclusion of breasts and experimentation with a variety of touches, such as with body oils, talcum powder, feathers, fabrics, and so on

3—As above but adding specific requests for preferred types of touch and the use of a back to front position to enable the person being touched to guide the partner's hand

Stage 2

1—Maintain the ban on intercourse but include genital touching as part of the established exercises, so no areas are now forbidden

2—While continuing all the above, concentrate more on the genitals to discover the sensations that result from different pressures in different areas

3—This is an optional stage for mutual masturbation to orgasm

Stage 3

1—While continuing all of the above and maintaining the ban on full intercourse,[1] the next step is containment without movement, allowing the penis to be accepted and contained by the vagina (modified for homosexual couples). Couples should progress at their preferred pace

2—Containment with gentle thrusting and rotating movement

3—Thrusting to orgasm

Physical remedies

Drug and surgical treatments are covered in later chapters.

Lubricants—Astroglyde generally is well tolerated by men and women and is available in high street stores, as are KY Jelly and Senselle. Carrier oils used in aromatherapy, such as peach kernel and sweet almond oils, can be excellent substitutes for patients who find water based lubricants to be an irritant or messy; **they must not be used with latex contraceptives, as the oil rots the rubber very fast and makes it ineffective**.

Tension rings—These are useful when an adequate erection can be obtained but not sustained. A tight rubber band at the base of the penis maintains an erection for up to 30 minutes.

Vacuum pumps—These promote an erection, which a tension ring then can sustain. Pumps are available in battery and manual forms.

Vibrators—These are available from sex shops and catalogues. The Viva Heat Massager is obtainable from department stores and large chemist shops and has the advantage of being useful in other contexts. It is mains operated, which may be a further advantage.

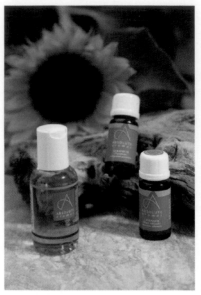

Carrier oils, as used in aromatherapy and massage, can be used as an alternative to water based lubricants for facilitating sexual intercourse

The picture of *Man, Woman and Fish* is reproduced with permission of Emily Young, courtesy of the Thackeray Gallery, London (private collection). The cartoon "Sam, the ceiling needs painting" is by Neville Spearman. The photograph of the couple lying in bed is reproduced with permission of Tony Stone. The engraving by Zichy is reproduced with permission of the Bridgeman Art Library Stapleton Collection. The photograph of the carrier oils is with permission of Absolute Aromas Limited, Hampshire. The photograph of the tension rings is with permission from Owen Mumford

1 Stanley E. Principles of managing sexual problems. *BMJ* 1981;282:1200-2
2 Masters WH, Johnson VE. *Human sexual inadequacy*. London: Churchill, 1970
3 Lieblum SR, Rosen RG (Eds). *Principles and practice of sex therapy*. Guildford: Guildford Press, 2000

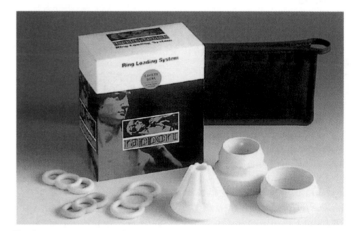

Tension rings can maintain an erection for up to 30 minutes when placed at the base of the penis

---

Further information

Most patients with sexual problems expect to be referred or at least investigated medically. It is very useful for the referrer to have some personal knowledge or contact with the next health care professional.

Lists of therapists can be obtained from:
- Institute of Psychosexual Medicine, 11 Chandos Street, London W1M 9DE (www.ipm.org.uk). This organisation also trains doctors in the practical skills of psychosexual medicine
- British Association for Sexual and Relationship Therapy, PO Box 13686, London SW20 9HZ (tel: 020 8543 2707; www.basrt.org.uk)
- Relate—Marriage Guidance, Herbert Gray College, Little Church Street, Rugby CV21 3AP (tel: 0845 456 1310; www.relate.org.uk). This organisation gives further specialised training in sexual therapy; a list of local centres can be obtained from its office
- British Association for Counselling and Psychotherapy, 1 Regent Place, Rugby, CV21 2PJ (tel: 01788 350899; www.counselling.co.uk)

Useful websites
- For women with vaginismus: Women's Therapy Center (www.womentc.com)
- For men with impotence (erectile dysfunction), retarded ejaculation and other sexual problems: The Sexual Dysfunction Association (formerly The Impotence Association) (tel: 0870 774 3571; www.impotence.org.uk), which gives a lot of information for patients
- Partner Therapy Group (tel: 07977 493667; www.partnertherapy.com)

Videos and DVDs
- *Sex, a lifelong pleasure* (a series of three videos). Great Dunmow: Press Play (tel: 01371 873138)
- *Lovers' guide* (a series introduced by Dr Andrew Stanway). London: Carlton Home Entertainment (tel: 020 8207 6207)
Both of these videos are 10 years old, but the information in the first of each scene is helpful

Books
- Zilbergeld B. *The new male sexuality*. London: Bantam, 1999
- Quilliam S. *A woman's complete illustrated guide to sex*. London: Fair Winds Press, 2003
- Litvinoff S. *Relate: sex in loving relationships*. London: Vermilion, 2001

---

2 Male anatomy, physiology, and behaviour

John M Tomlinson

Many adult men (and a large number of women) are ignorant of the structure and function of the male sexual organs, even though the penis is used for micturition and boys become accustomed to handling their genitalia from an early age. It is important to be clear on their structure and function, particularly if helping with sexual problems to clarify misapprehensions and myths (see Chapter 9 for anatomy and physiology of sexual function).

Anatomy and physiology

The penis

The penis consists of two parallel corpora cavernosa (cavernous bodies) in line with the corpus spongiosum (spongy body), which encircles the urethra on the underside of the penis and expands at its tip to form the glans. Proximally, the corpora cavernosa are attached to the pelvis just anterior to the ischial tuberosities. A thick fascia, Buck's fascia, binds the three together and is covered in turn by the superficial or Colles fascia. The trabecular structure of the corpora consists of smooth muscle and fibroelastic tissue; the muscle relaxes on sexual arousal, causing the penis to become erect with incoming blood. Over all of this is the very loose and mobile penile skin that allows the penis to expand during erection.

The glans—The glans surrounds the urethral meatus and consists entirely of corpus spongiosum. It has a large concentration of sensory nerve endings from the pudendal nerves, particularly around the coronal rim and underneath at the frenulum, the thin fold of skin that attaches the glans to the foreskin.

The foreskin—In most uncircumcised men, the glans pushes out from the encircling foreskin to a varying extent during sexual arousal. In a small proportion of young men, the frenulum is tight, which may cause bowing of the end of the penis on erection or even difficulty in retracting the foreskin. Generally, it stretches in use, but it sometimes rips during intercourse, with much bleeding and anguish for the man and his partner. If the frenulum causes problems, it can easily be snipped in a general practitioner's treatment room.

Circumcision—In a recent large survey in the United Kingdom, 21.9% of all men, including Jewish and Muslim men, had been circumcised, but this varied with age.[1] Only 12.5% of men aged 16-24 years were circumcised compared with 32.3% of those aged 45-59 years, which probably reflects changing public health policies from the 1940s.

As the penis varies markedly in appearance from one man to another—in colour, length, girth, shape, and presence of a foreskin—its size and shape can cause considerable worry to its owner. The length of the flaccid penis is 5-9.5 cm. The erect penis varies much less in size than generally is believed, and the normal range is 12.5-17.5 cm,[2] with an average of 16 cm. The distal girth (measured just proximal to the glans) averages 12 cm.

Teenagers often worry about the size of their penis. This is perpetuated by men not appreciating that temperature has a large effect and by not realising that a smaller penis enlarges by a greater percentage volume than a larger flaccid penis, that magazine photographs are angled carefully, that especially well endowed "actors" or models are chosen for videos, and that, most importantly of all, when a man looks down he sees a foreshortened view of himself.

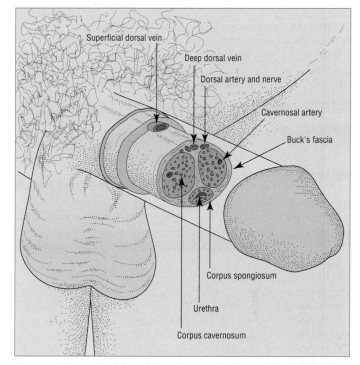

Anatomy of the penis. Adapted from *Impotence* by Foster MC and Cole M with permission of Schwarz Pharma

Uncircumcising*

A doctor who had been circumcised as a child had had minor discomfort in his glans for years, so that he always wore tight supportive underwear to minimise friction. He noticed that the glans had remarkably little sensitivity but assumed that little could be done about it until he read a book on uncircumcising (J Bigelow's *The joy of uncircumcising!* Antioch, IL: Hourglass Books, 1992).

He decided to refashion his foreskin and stretched the penile skin with weights and surgical tape. After 10 days, he was more comfortable than he had ever been, and, after 10 weeks, intercourse was easier and frictionless. He continued and was delighted, and he concluded that doctors and medical students need to be taught that the foreskin has a function and is as important to the penis as the eyelid to the eye—a protector, moistener, and sensitiser—and he advocated conservatism, especially in treating phimosis.

* Story taken from Personal view: The joy of uncircumcising. *BMJ* 1994;309:676-7

An 80 year old man, on being given a test dose of alprostadil for erectile dysfunction, was delighted to be told that his feeling of shame at his small penis for the past 65 years was completely unjustified and that his size was well within the normal range

Erections larger than 20 cm in white men are unusual, and claims have to be taken with a pinch of salt. The only way to make the penis look longer is by cutting the suspensory ligament, which lets it dangle but destabilises it, and most surgeons fight shy of doing this. The girth can be increased by injecting abdominal fat around the shaft, but this seems to degenerate into lumpy nodules after a few months.

Spontaneous erections occur often in young men, especially in their teenage years. At times, these can be extremely embarrassing, especially as, at first, they may not be aware of it happening and because it may have nothing to do with sexual arousal. Fortunately, this acute sensitivity occurs less often with time.

The scrotum

The scrotum varies in external appearance under different circumstances. In young people, during cold weather, exercise, and the excitement and plateau phases of sexual stimulation, the subcutaneous dartos muscle contracts and the scrotal skin is corrugated and closely applied to the testes. In warmth, under loose clothing, and in older men, the scrotum hangs elongated and flaccid, which allows a decrease in temperature of up to 1.0°C; this is believed to enhance sperm production.

The testes

The testes measure about 5 × 2.5 × 2.5 cm, although they can vary in size from day to day in the same person, and the left usually hangs lower than the right. Production of spermatozoa and testosterone are under the control of the hypothalamus, which produces gonadotrophin releasing hormone (GnRH). This in turn controls the pituitary's release of luteinising hormone (LH), which is responsible for production of testosterone, and follicle stimulating hormone (FSH), which stimulates production of spermatozoa and oestrogen.

Spermatozoa travel from the seminiferous tubules to the seminal vesicles, where up to 70% of the total ejaculate is formed; the rest of the ejaculate is produced by the prostate, is first to be ejaculated, and contains the highest concentration of sperm. Although the seminal vesicles are said not to store sperms, despite their name, no one has identified clearly where the sperms found in the first 10-20 ejaculates after vasectomy are stored.

Semen usually is thick and sticky immediately after ejaculation, but it rapidly liquefies. This leads some patients to think erroneously that the quality of their sperm has diminished or become "thin."

Cowper's glands—These two subprostatic, paraurethral, pea sized glands produce a clear, slightly sticky fluid at the penile meatus on sexual arousal. This varies in quantity from a bead to 5 ml, although some men may not be aware of it at all. Colloquially known as pre-come (or pre-cum), it seems to be a natural lubricant and may contain a few live spermatozoa.

The breasts

Men have only a very small amount of breast tissue, but, at puberty, one or other breast may enlarge and become painful, causing acute embarrassment to the adolescent. This gynaecomastia usually settles within a year or so, but, rarely, it may be severe enough to warrant a breast reduction. Carcinoma of the adult male breast can occur, but it is uncommon, occurring in about one in 1200 men.

Non-genital erogenous zones

These include the mouth, skin, anus, and rectum. The anus is highly sensitive, and insertion of a finger or other object (including a penis) is not uncommon in heterosexual

> A 20 year old undergraduate, after enjoying his first sexual encounter, was mortified and humiliated the next day to hear that his partner had told all his friends (men and women) how small and poorly endowed he was genitally. He became completely impotent until he was seen in an erectile dysfunction clinic. After treatment with alprostadil, he was shown with a tape measure that he was actually at the upper level of the normal range of length and girth. He recovered full function

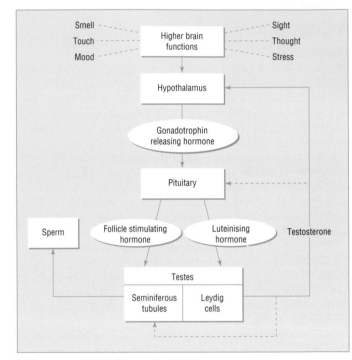

Endocrine regulation of sperm production

Assessing endocrine function

- A low concentration of testosterone in the serum often leads to reduced sexual interest and erectile dysfunction, but many men can perform normally
- Serum testosterone concentration alone is not a reliable guide
- The free androgen index (currently the nearest equivalent to a measure of the biologically available testosterone) is a better guide and is found by dividing the concentration of testosterone in serum by the concentration of serum hormone binding globulin (SHBG), expressed as a percentage
- Most authorities would treat with replacement testosterone if the free androgen index is much less than 50% of the age related normal range, although a level as low as 35% is accepted by many as still normal
- To try and exclude carcinoma of the prostrate before giving replacement testosterone is essential. Digital rectal examination and serum prostatic specific antigen (PSA) concentration should be done in all prospective recipients (see Chapter 19)
- A high luteinising hormone (LH) concentration suggests that the interstitial, or Leydig, cells, which manufacture testosterone, are not responding
- A low luteinising hormone concentration may indicate that the pituitary is not producing enough

intercourse, as well as homosexual intercourse. In a survey of British couples in 2001, 12.3% of men and 11.3% of women had had anal intercourse in the previous year—almost double the number in 1990 (see Chapter 13).[3]

Puberty

The obvious physical changes of puberty in boys occur a year or so later than in girls, with an adolescent growth spurt, on average, at age 14 years. The earliest physical change is in the growth of the testes as a result of production of testosterone through the stimulation of luteinising hormone. Boys begin to undergo genital development at an average age of 11 years 6 months, with the genitals reaching adult size and shape by an average of 14 years 9 months. Some boys develop rapidly over a year, whereas others can take five years.[4]

As testosterone production increases, the penis, prostate, and seminal vesicles grow. As soon as enough testosterone is present for them to function, ejaculation is possible; this occurs, on average, at the age of twelve and a half. Production of sperm starts in childhood and becomes fully established when, or soon after, ejaculation is possible. The youngest recorded father of a child in the United Kingdom in modern times was an 11 year old boy who claimed in 1997 to have made a 14 year old girl pregnant. A healthy baby was born in January 1998.[5]

Hair starts to develop on the pubis with the start of genital growth at age 11 years; growth of axillary hair follows some 12-24 months later. Growth of chest hair may start during puberty or later, and may continue to grow for 10 years or more. Deepening of the voice is caused by testosterone stimulation of the larynx, which lengthens anteriorly. The average age at which voice change occurs now is 13.5 years compared with age 18 years in 1750.[6]

Nocturnal and early morning erections are a normal part of paradoxical or rapid eye movement sleep (and are not connected with having a full bladder). A 13 year old boy will have, on average, four erections a night and, for about a third of his time sleeping, will have penile tumescence. This rate falls slowly to two or more erections, occupying a fifth of sleeping time, in men in their 60s. Nocturnal emissions ("wet dreams") seem to be a physiological safety valve and occur in more than 80% of men at some time, with two thirds of 17 year old boys having at least one a month unless ejaculation with masturbation or intercourse is regular.[8] A rapid decline in nocturnal emissions follows, so that few men over the age of 30 years continue to have them.

Sexual intercourse
The proportion of boys in Britain who have sexual intercourse before the age of 16 years has increased to a sizeable minority (29.9% in 2000[9]). The median age rises with the level of education and with those from the Indian subcontinent, but a much larger proportion of black boys than white boys start intercourse before the age of 16 years. The main factors that tempt boys to start include spur of the moment action (44.2%) and curiosity (40.5%).[1]

Sexual arousal and response

Masters and Johnson discovered the four stages of sexual response in men.[7] Most information comes from their work in the 1960s and 1970s.

Stage 1: excitement phase
This results from physical or psychological stimulation, or both, which can rapidly lead to erection of the penis and drawing up

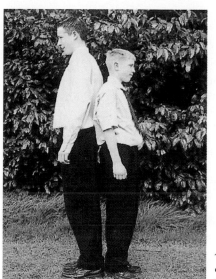

Two boys aged 14.3 years developing at different rates (180 and 165 cm tall)

Masturbation now is seen as a perfectly healthy form of sexual expression, and fortunately it no longer is regarded as dirty and sinful, as it used to be when religious authority saw it as a threat to health and morality (as many men from southeast Asia are still taught). Estimates are that 95% of men have masturbated, and the frequency seems to vary from daily to once a month, with the highest incidence in the teenage years and early 20s, depending on other sexual activities[7]

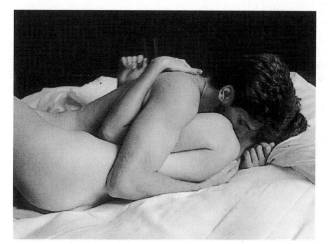

The main factors that tempt boys are spur of the moment action and curiosity

of the testes (for detailed pharmacology of the response, see Chapter 9). The corpora fill with blood from the helicine arteries via the internal iliac and pudendal arteries.

Stage 2: plateau stage

The diameter of the glans increases and deepens in colour with vasocongestion, which also causes the testes to grow up to 50% larger than normal. The testes continue to rise and a feeling of perineal warmth occurs. The buttocks and thighs tighten, the heart rate increases, respiration is quicker, and blood pressure rises slightly. Orgasm is imminent.

Stage 3: orgasm and ejaculation

These are different processes that can be impaired selectively, but they generally are taken to be synonymous (colloquially called "coming" or "climax"). The vas deferens, prostate, and seminal vesicles begin a series of contractions that force semen into the bulb of the urethra—the so called brink of control, when ejaculation cannot be stopped—and then contractions of the prostate and pelvic floor muscles lead to ejaculation. The rectal sphincter and the neck of the bladder tighten, while the contractions force the semen out.

Stage 4: resolution

After ejaculation, a refractory or recovery time occurs, when further orgasm is not possible. Recovery time varies from a few minutes to many hours, or even a couple of days in elderly men. (Some religious groups, such as Taoists, claim that men, as well as women, can achieve multiple orgasms). Detumescence now occurs, and the changes of stage 1 reverse, with the addition of heavy fast respiration, tachycardia, and sometimes profuse sweating. Sexual arousal without orgasm can lead to resolution being slower, with pelvic fullness and penile and testicular aching of varying intensity because of vasocongestion.

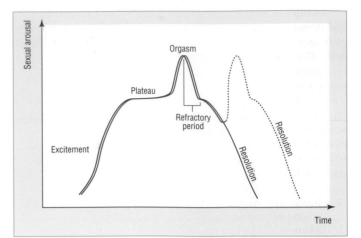

The sexual response cycle in men. Dotted line shows possibility of second orgasm and ejaculation after the refractory period. Adapted from Master WH, Johnson VE. *Human sexual response.* Boston, MA: Little, Brown, 1966

> Orgasms vary at different times in the same person and from person to person, depending on circumstances—mood, partner, occasion, frequency

> A partial or even full erection may sometimes be maintained during the recovery period, especially in younger men

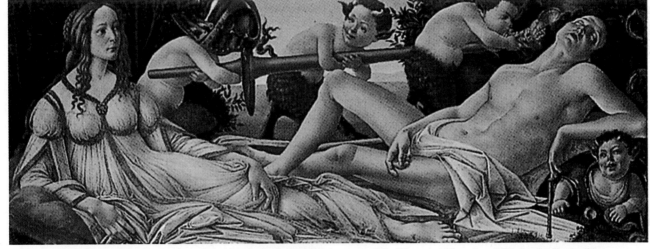

After ejaculation the man experiences a recovery period when further orgasm is not possible (*Venus and Mars*, circa 1485, Sandro Botticelli)

The effects of age

Sexual ability and drive continue well into old age, although a decline in frequency of activity is seen. This can be partially explained by poorer health, but also results in part from cultural expectations.

Men aged over 55 years usually take longer and need more direct manual or oral stimulation for the penis to become erect than younger men, tend to have less firm erections, produce a smaller amount of semen, and have less intense ejaculations. They usually have less physical need to ejaculate, a longer refractory period, and reduced muscle tension.[7]

> A decrease in frequency of sexual activity can be partially explained by poorer health, but also results in part from cultural expectations

An older man with erectile dysfunction is often humiliated and demoralised when his doctor says, "What can you expect at your age?" and fear of this dissuades many from asking for help. They can be reassured by the results of a global study of men aged 70-80 years, in which 53% had had sexual intercourse in the past 12 months and 20% had intercourse at least five times a month.[10] The importance attached to regular intercourse in younger days correlates significantly with sexual activity in old age. The adage "If you don't use it, you lose it" has more than a grain of truth, and obviously there is no reason to doubt that men (and women) can (and do) enjoy sexual activity to a ripe old age.

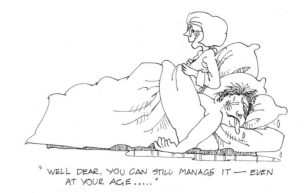

" WELL DEAR, YOU CAN STILL MANAGE IT — EVEN AT YOUR AGE ....."

1 Johnson AM, Wadsworth J, Wellings K, Field F. *Sexual attitudes and lifestyles*. Oxford: Blackwell Scientific, 1994
2 Dickinson RL. *Human sex anatomy*. London: Krieger Publishing, 1971. In Coxon APM. *Between the sheets: project SIGMA*. London: Cassell, 1996
3 Wellings K, Nanchahal K, Macdowall W, McManus S, Erens B, Mercer CH et al. Sexual behaviour in Britain: early heterosexual experience. *Lancet* 2001;358:1843-50
4 Marshall WA, Tanner JM. Variation in the pubertal changes in boys. *Arch Dis Child* 1970;45:13-23
5 *Daily Telegraph* 1998, Jan 21
6 Grumbach M. The neuroendocrinology of puberty. *Hosp Pract* 1980;Mar:51-60
7 Masters WH, Johnson VE, Kolodny RC. *Human sexuality*. New York: Harper Collins, 1995
8 Bancroft J. *Human sexuality and its problems*. Edinburgh: Churchill Livingstone, 1989
9 Wellings K, Nanchahal K, Macdowall W, McManus S, Erens B, Mercer CH et al. Sexual behaviour in Britain: early sexual experience. *Lancet* 2001;358:1843-50
10 Gingell C, Nicolosi A, Glasser DB, Brock G, Burat J for the global study of sexual attitudes and behaviour. Sexual behaviours and functioning in mature men: results of an international study (in press)

Further reading

- Masters WH, Johnson VE, Kolodny RC. *Human sexuality*. 5th ed. New York: Harper Collins, 1995. Useful for an authoritative (American) view of sex.
- Godson S. *The sex book*. London: Cassell, 2002. Very readable, informative, authoritative and up to date (British) view of sex. Ideal to recommend to patients.

The figure of endocrine regulation of sperm production is adapted from Masters WH, Johnson VE, Kolodny RC. *Human sexuality*. New York: Harper Collins, 1995. The figure of the sexual response cycle in men is adapted from Masters WH, Johnson VE. *Human sexual response*. Boston, MA: Little Brown, 1966. The painting by Botticelli is reproduced with permission of Bridgeman Art Library. The photograph of the two boys is reproduced with their and their parents' permission. The cartoon "You can still manage it..." is reproduced with permission of Tony Goffe.

3 Female sexual anatomy, physiology, and behaviour

Tony Parsons

Puberty

Functional adult sexual anatomy and physiology are established during the course of puberty. This process, which is spread over several years, consists of a series of overlapping developments, including growth and development of the breasts, growth of pubic and axillary hair, accelerated growth in height, and, finally, menstruation and ovulation. The age at which each stage is reached varies widely, such that one girl may have completed the process at an age when another has not even started.

Early menstrual cycles usually are irregular, and ovulation may take one to two years to be established after the first period. During this time, the womb lining is being built up and shed in response to changes in oestrogen levels only. Once ovulation begins, the production of progesterone in the corpus luteum controls the timing of the cycles, but this also triggers the process that leads to dysmenorrhoea.

Although there has been a gradual trend for menarche to occur at a younger age during this century, this only partially explains the reduction in age of first sexual experience and first sexual intercourse. A recent British survey found that 25.6% of girls had started intercourse before the age of 16 years (compared with 29.9% of men),[1] whereas 40 years ago, it was fewer than 1%.

Sexual anatomy

The external genitalia, or vulva, consist of the mons veneris, the labia, the clitoris, and the perineum. All are innervated heavily with sensory nerve fibres and are involved in the physiological processes of sexual response. The mons veneris is particularly sensitive to touch or pressure sensation. The labia are an important source of sexual sensation for most women, and the labia minora have a spongy core that becomes engorged on arousal. The clitoris consists of the clitoral glans and shaft, which are covered by the clitoral hood. The clitoris itself is highly sensitive to touch, pressure, and temperature, and it is subject to indirect stimulation during intercourse by the movement of the labia minora. Bartholin's glands, which lie posteriorly within the labia minora, were thought to be responsible for vaginal lubrication, but they now are considered of minor importance.

Many people, especially men, do not realise that the vagina has few sensory nerve endings except at the introitus, and, therefore, the inner two thirds of the vagina are relatively insensitive. In non-parous women, the average lengths of the posterior and anterior walls are 7.5 cm and 6 cm, respectively. The concept of the G (Grafenburg) spot, a particularly sensitive region in the front wall of the vagina midway between the pubic bone and the cervix,[2] remains controversial and has not been proved scientifically. The cervix itself is highly variable in its sensitivity and often plays no role in sexual enjoyment.

Many other parts of the body, as well as those involved in reproduction, are potential sources of sexual arousal. The insides of the thigh, the neck, and the perineum often are erogenous zones, as is the mouth, including the lips and tongue. The anal canal and perianal area also are highly sensitive to touch, and anal stimulation or intercourse can be part of normal heterosexual activity.

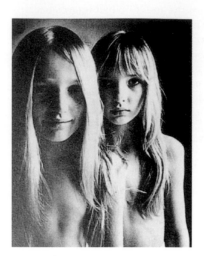

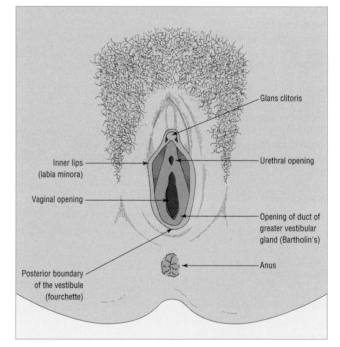

Female genitalia with labia parted. Redrawn from Banfield J. *Human sexuality and its problems.* Edinburgh: Churchill Livingstone, 1989

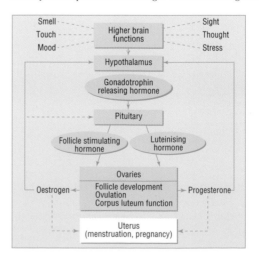

Endocrine regulation of sexual development in women

Physiology of sexual response

A physiological sexual response requires intact pelvic innervation, adequate local blood supply, and a normal hormonal environment. Sexual arousal can occur under a wide variety of situations and may be triggered purely by cerebral events or response to physical contact. Excitement, however, is not linked invariably to arousal. It is possible for women under some circumstances to show the physiological changes of arousal without experiencing any of the pleasurable sensations normally associated with this. Episodes of vaginal lubrication also occur during sleep (in the same way as nocturnal erections in men) and are not controlled by the specific content of dreams.

Our understanding of the sexual response cycle is based largely on Masters and Johnson's original observations and assumes that their sample of volunteer participants was representative of the full range of normal physiology.[3] Their classification divides sexual response into four phases: excitement, plateau, orgasm, and resolution. The phases represent an incremental increase in sexual excitement, and each is a necessary precursor for the next phase. It has been suggested that an extra phase normally precedes these; this is the desire phase, the part of sexual response that is perhaps the least understood.

Excitement or arousal phase

This is the initial response to sexual stimulation and, like each phase, has genital and systemic components. The reflex of vasodilatation within the genitalia is mediated through two centres in the spinal cord (one at the level of T11-L2, the other at S2-S4) and through specific receptors in the pelvic smooth muscle. Increased blood flow in the vaginal wall results in a transudate through the vaginal walls, which is the main source of lubrication. At the same time, the inner two thirds of the vagina balloon out or "tent," and the vulva becomes engorged.

The systemic component of this phase includes increases in pulse and respiratory rates and blood pressure. Some women also show general vasocongestion, especially over the upper torso and neck. The excitement phase is vulnerable to interruption by distraction: internally, such as by extraneous thoughts, or by interruption.

Plateau phase

This is sometimes regarded as part of arousal and represents a consolidation of the changes that occurred during the excitement phase. Congestion in the outer third of the vagina reaches a maximum, producing a firm area of engorged tissue around the introitus (the so called "orgasmic platform"). Breast changes also reach a maximum in this phase: breast size may increase by 20-25% in many women who have not breast fed, and the areolae become congested, so that the nipple looks less erect. Finally, as orgasm approaches, the clitoris becomes firmly retracted against the pubic bone and seems to disappear. Although described as a plateau, this phase actually requires continuous stimulation to build up sexual excitement to the intensity that is needed for orgasm.

Orgasm

Objectively, orgasm is a peak of pleasurable sensation and the release of sexual tension that has built up during the preceding phases, together with involuntary rhythmic contraction of the genital muscles (at 0.8 second intervals). Subjectively, orgasms differ widely in description from one woman to another and from one occasion to another, although descriptions of orgasms by men and by women are remarkably similar. The importance of orgasm for sexual satisfaction may also vary. After orgasm,

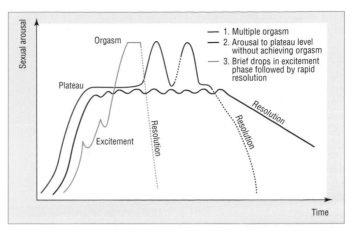

Sexual response cycle in women. Redrawn from Masters WH, Johnson VE. *Human sexual response.* Boston, MA: Little Brown, 1996

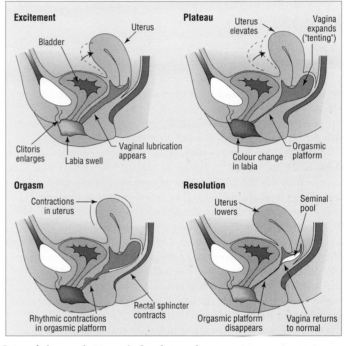

Internal changes that occur in female sexual response

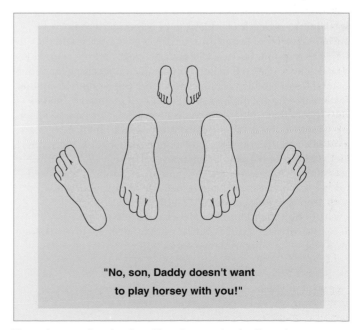

"No, son, Daddy doesn't want to play horsey with you!"

The excitement phase is vulnerable to interruption by distraction most women do not have the refractory period that is seen in men, and further stimulation can produce further orgasms.

The nature of the orgasm clearly is not affected by the type of stimulation used to produce it, although masturbatory orgasms may be somewhat more intense. Many men, and women, do not realise that fewer than one in three women can reach a climax from intercourse alone and that foreplay, such as stimulation of the clitoris (manually or orally) and touching and caressing other erogenous zones, is essential for orgasm to occur in most women.

Resolution

After orgasm, the body gradually returns to the non-aroused state. In older, parous women, impairment of this resolution phase, especially if associated with high levels of arousal and failure to climax, may lead to pelvic congestion with non-specific symptoms of aching in the lower back and pelvis, which has its exact counterpart in men.

Menopause

The menopause may have an impact on women's sexuality in three main ways.

Psychologically, it may represent a watershed and a point beyond which a woman feels she no longer can, or should, be sexually attractive.

Physical symptoms, particularly severe night sweats and mood swings, can be highly disruptive to a sexual relationship.

Oestrogen deficiency causes specific physical responses in some women. These include a failure of vaginal lubrication (this may start before the actual cessation of periods), development of vaginal dryness and irritation, reduced sensation in the vulval tissues, and impaired neural transmission of these sensations.

Painful uterine contractions at orgasm seem to be more common after the menopause. The natural loss of collagen may result in the vagina becoming less elastic, particularly in those who are not sexually active. The vaginal introitus and the surrounding vulva may atrophy. Long term oestrogen replacement (as a local cream or vaginal tablet, or even systemically) may be needed to prevent or reverse these changes. Chapter 19 gives an up to date survey of this subject.

Sexual drive

Sexual drive is clearly complex but poorly understood. A hormonal element probably underlies sexual interest and the ability to respond, but no clear patterns exist, and response to sexual activity may well depend on complex underlying emotional factors. Considerable variation exists from one woman to another, particularly during the menstrual cycle and pregnancy. Studies have shown that women who have a less satisfactory sexual life or are unable to discuss their sexuality openly with their partner are most likely to experience a reduction in sexual satisfaction when they pass through a time of physiological change. Sexual drive actually may improve at the menopause, but when it is reduced (either as a primary problem or because of vaginal dryness), oestrogen replacement often is highly effective.

Although the general tendency is for sexual drive to decrease with age (and duration of relationship), no upper age limits exist for a happy active sexual life.

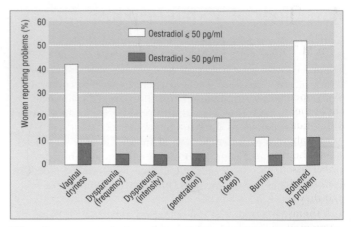

Effect of serum concentrations of oestradiol on reported sexual problems in postmenopausal women. Adapted from Sarrel P. Sexuality and menopause. *J Obstet Gynaecol* 1990;75:265-355

Symptoms associated with urogenital ageing

- Vaginal dryness
- Vaginal irritation
- Dyspareunia
- Post-coital bleeding
- Urinary frequency and urgency

Effects of oestrogen deficiency on sexual response

- Vaginal blood flow decreases
- Vaginal secretions decrease
- pH increased
- Blood flow to clitoris and labia diminished
- Sensory neurological impairment

Sex in pregnancy

- Physiology remains essentially the same
- Erogenous zones may alter
- Preferred stimulation may alter
- Different positions may be needed for comfortable intercourse

---

1 Wellings K, Nanchahal K, Macdowall W, McManus S, Erens B, Mercer CH et al. Sexual behaviour in Britain: early heterosexual experience. *Lancet* 2001;358:1843-50
2 Grafenburg E. The role of the urethra in the female orgasm. *Int J Sexology* 1950;3:145-8
3 Masters WH, Johnson VE. *Human sexual response*. Boston: Little, Brown, 1966

The figures of endocrine regulation of sexual development and internal changes during female sexual response are adapted from Masters WH, Johnson VE, Kolodny RC. *Human sexuality*. New York: Harper Collins, 1995. The female sexual response cycle is adapted from Masters WH, Johnson VE. *Human sexual response*. Boston MA: Little, Brown, 1966. The effect of serum oestradiol on sexual problems is adapted from Sarrel P. Sexuality and menopause. *J Obstet Gynaecol* 1990;75: 265-355. All figures are used with the publishers' permission. The cartoon "No, Son …" is by Neville Spearman, 1966.

4 Taking a sexual history

John M Tomlinson

Many doctors, nurses, and medical students are concerned about their ability to take an appropriate history from a patient with sexual problems. The main difference between taking a history about a sexual problem and an ordinary medical history is that the patient (and often the doctor) commonly is embarrassed and uncomfortable. Patients may feel ashamed or even humiliated at having to ask for help with sexual problems that they think are private and that they should be able to cope with themselves. This is true particularly with men, especially young men, who have to admit to erectile dysfunction and, as they see it, the loss of their masculinity. Some hospital doctors get over this initial difficulty by giving patients a preconsultation questionnaire. Many patients like this, but a substantial number dislike its anonymity and apparent coldness.

As with other history taking, the doctor must consider how to put the patient at ease, find out the real problem, discover the patient's background and clinical history, and work out a plan of management with the patient. The doctor should try to avoid showing embarrassment, especially if the patient wants to talk about things that are outside the doctor's experience, as this can cause the patient to clam up.

Above all, sufficient time must be allowed: 45-60 minutes is an ideal that unfortunately often is not possible to achieve, although in general practice, the patient can be asked to come back for a longer appointment at another time. Much can be achieved, however, in 10-15 minutes.

Making patients feel comfortable

If the doctor's attitude is matter of fact, then the patient also will relax and become matter of fact. Whatever the patient admits to, the doctor must be non-judgmental.

A patient's approach to the problem often is tentative and hidden by euphemisms: statements such as "I think I need a check up" or "By the way, I am itchy/sore/have a discharge down below." These comments may be slipped into a consultation about some other problem, and the doctor must decide whether to investigate the matter immediately or persuade the patient to return for a longer consultation.

Various interview techniques can be used to help patients relax more quickly; most are used by many doctors intuitively. These include the manner of greeting a patient, seeing that the patient is seated comfortably, and ensuring privacy and freedom from interruption (especially in a hospital clinic). A seat placed at the side of the desk provides a greater opportunity to observe the patient's body language, as well as being a more friendly arrangement.

Useful observations on patients' body language include:

- Their use of hands and arms, such as uneasily twiddling with rings, defensive arm crossing, or protective holding of a bag or briefcase on a lap
- A pectoral flush seen to creep over the upper chest and neck in women, as well as some men (now that fewer men wear buttoned up shirts); this indicates unease despite an outward appearance of calm
- The body's position in the chair—depressed slump, tautly sitting bolt upright, or relaxed sprawl
- Postural echo, when doctor and patient sit in mirror images of each other's position; when this is adopted, harmony and empathy exists between the speakers.

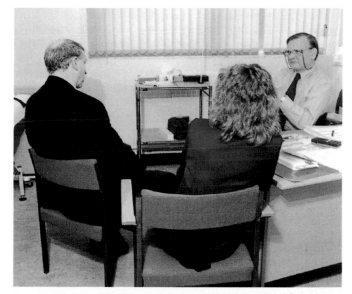

Seats placed at the side of the desk make a more friendly arrangement for an interview and it is easier to observe a couple's body language to each other, which gives clues to their relationship

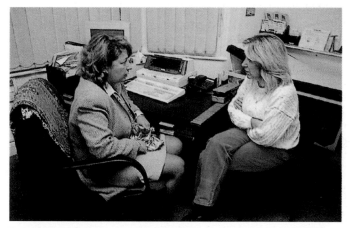

Patients' body language, such as defensive crossing of arms, can show their state of mind

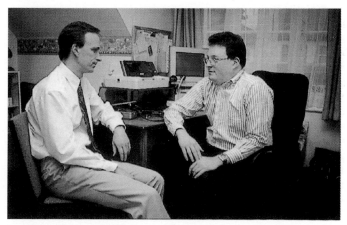

Postural echo, when doctor and patient sit in mirror image of each other's position, indicates empathy between the speakers

Finding out the problem

When people talk about embarrassing subjects, they often are vague and circumlocutory, and what they are trying to say must be clarified. Words such as "impotence," for example, can mean different things to different men (and their partners), including failure to get an erection, failure to maintain an erection, and premature ejaculation. Equally, a phrase such as "I'm sore down below" can mean anything from pruritus ani to some anatomical problem such as prolapse or genital warts.

Careful and tactful elucidation is needed, and vagueness must be clarified. The questioner has to be particularly sharp in picking up what the patient is trying to say and be relaxed and unfazed by the subject matter, but this can be overdone.

Very early in the discussion, the patient must be assured of complete confidentiality, particularly with respect to practice and hospital clinic staff, especially if personal secrets are disclosed, such as extramarital affairs. A number of factors should be noted during the interview.

Choice of terminology

One issue that worries many doctors is whether to use vernacular terms in discussions because of their emotional charge, and some veer to the safety of using only medical terms. Patients also may try to express their problem in medical terms, because of embarrassment about using colloquialisms and fear of causing offence, but they may well get the meaning wrong. This can cause problems in getting an accurate history, but doctors must use very careful judgment to decide if it would be more appropriate to use the language of the streets.

Although frank articles are published in many magazines and newspapers, many patients, especially younger women, still will not know the meaning of "orgasm" but will understand "come." Fellatio and cunnilingus are not words in general use, and use of the street versions would assume a very relaxed and empathic discussion, but "oral sex" is acceptable to men and women of all ages as an alternative. Usually, the line is very fine and often is related to age and sex.

Open questions

The way in which open and closed questions are used in history taking is crucial. A closed question expects a specific reply, such as "Yes" or "No," and is characteristic of the medical model of history taking, such as: "Have you had this problem before? Does it hurt when you pass water? Did you practise safe sex?"

Starting with an open question—"How can I help you?"— and continuing with open questions—"What's the problem?" or "What do you think caused the difficulty?"—gives patients an opportunity to expand and to say what is really bothering them. Many younger doctors are worried that a garrulous person might get out of hand, but remaining in control is a skill a good interviewer learns quickly. Judgmental questions—"Don't you think you're past that sort of thing now?"—should be avoided.

Silence

Silence is a powerful tool in taking a good history, and the best interviewers—whether on the radio, on television, or in the consulting room—have realised this. However, many doctors find it extremely difficult not to end a silence, speaking prematurely because they are embarrassed by the quiet or feel that it is rude not to say anything, whereas the patient is often using the time to order his or her thoughts. Valuable details may be lost if those thoughts are cut across by an inappropriate statement from the doctor. The rule is, have patience.

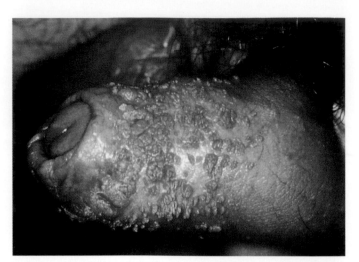

Phrases such as, "I'm sore below" can mean anything from minor irritation to genital warts

A patient went back to a general practitioner's receptionist to make a new appointment and said, "I don't want to see him again. I only went in with a cold and he asked me all about my sex life."

Factors to be noted during interview

- The patient's marital state
- How many previous sexual partners the patient has had and which sex (do not be afraid to ask men outright if they have ever had sex with another man)
- Who the current partner is and for how long
- How many children the patient has and which of the children lives with the patient
- Whether there is obvious stress in the family
- Whether there are financial worries

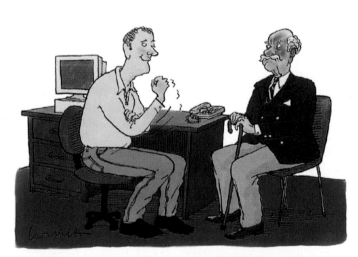

Doctors must use very careful judgment when deciding if it would be appropriate to use colloquialisms when discussing a sexual problem

A 16 year old boy was struggling to find medical words to explain his anxieties about masturbation and ejaculation. When the doctor tried to help him out by using colloquial terms the boy looked startled and then grinned and said, "I didn't know doctors knew those words." The rest of the consultation was much more relaxed and informative

Repetition

Repetition of the last word or phrase in a sentence, especially one that is loaded emotionally, is a powerful technique that can be used to get a patient to elaborate on what they are trying to say. Everyone uses this technique in everyday life, often without thinking, but when used deliberately without overtones—although it may seem artificial and forced—it can elicit much useful information.

Content of a sexual history

Although a joint interview always is much more valuable, patients often prefer to discuss things alone in the first instance. A warm invitation for the partner, coupled with the observation that a sexual problem is not the patient's problem alone, can put the patient's anxieties into perspective. To be complete, the history must include several factors.

Social history

A detailed social history helps to put the patient into context. The patient's problem can be the first item to be discussed, but taking a social and medical history before exploring the problem allows the patient time to relax while talking about familiar things such as children, home, and job and enables the doctor to put the problems into perspective. Even if the doctor is the patient's general practitioner and knows him or her well, a review of the social history will give a valuable update and incidental information that is often highly relevant.

Medical history

It used to be thought that all sexual problems, especially erectile dysfunction, were psychogenic in origin. General opinion has shifted to accept that a large proportion can have a physical basis, although, not surprisingly, often with a psychogenic overlay. To take a detailed medical history, particularly bearing in mind illnesses that may affect sexual performance, is therefore important.

Physical causes of sexual problems

Condition	Effect
Diabetes	Can eventually cause impotence in up to half of affected men
Depression and psychotic illnesses	Cause loss of sexual desire (but not necessarily loss of function) in a high proportion of both men and women, but careful questioning is needed to elicit them Altered sleep pattern, especially early waking, is a valuable indicator of depression
Heart disease	Accounts for erectile dysfunction in many men, especially when combined with hyperlipidaemia and arteriopathy
Operations and trauma	Especially gynaecological and prostate operations and trauma, can cause problems Damage to the pelvis or spine is another obvious cause. Many men find that they cannot get an erection after major cardiac surgery
Prolactinoma	Rarely, may present as a loss of sexual desire and headaches in younger men
Other hormone deficiencies	Such as thyroid and testosterone reduce sexual desire and performance in both sexes Often, the symptoms of lack of testosterone mimic those of depression
Pain	For example, of arthritis, vaginal atrophy in the older woman, or a phimosis, can be very offputting to one or other partner

Example of using repetition to elicit information

"Doctor, I think I need a check up"
"Yes, of course. It's quite a time since the last one. Let me start with your blood pressure…"
Compare this with
"Doctor, I think I need a check up."
"Check up?"
"Yes, I'm not performing as well as I used to."
"Performing?"
"Yes, well, you know, I think I'm impotent. My wife is very good about it and doesn't complain, but I feel so guilty and ashamed."
"Ashamed?"
"I feel terrible. I don't feel a man any more, especially as we used to have such a good sex life…"

Questions to be asked in a sexual history

- The problem as the patient sees it
- How long has the problem been present?
- Is the problem related to the time, place, or partner?
- Is there a loss of sex drive or dislike of sexual contact?
- Are there problems in the relationship?
- What are the stress factors as seen by the patient and by the partner?
- Is there other anxiety, guilt, or anger not expressed?
- Are there physical problems such as pain felt by either partner?

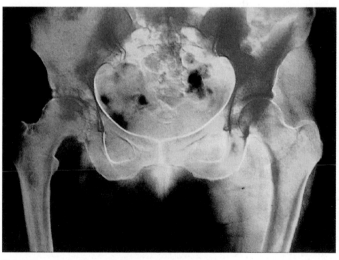

Painful osteoarthritis of the hips or knees that limits movement can be very inhibiting for sexual activity

Patient's (and partner's) view of the problem

Assessment of a couple's relationship just by looking at their body language to each other is useful. Marital dysfunction or simply sexual boredom after many years together can be a major cause of impotence.

In men with erectile dysfunction, the patient's, and especially his partner's, views of the causes are helpful, as this often shows their anxieties about other problems, including malignancy. It is also useful to know the speed of onset: organic causes such as diabetes tend to result in slow development of sexual problems, whereas psychogenic problems appear more rapidly, although this guide is not infallible. A psychogenic reason for the problem is indicated if the man gets erections during the night or on early waking or if he can masturbate successfully—although many are reluctant to admit this in front of their partner. (Erectile dysfunction is covered in Chapter 12.)

Strict upbringing and religious beliefs, especially if there is disparity between the partners, as in mixed marriages, can often have a devastating effect on a sexual relationship. Other questions include whether unemployment or the threat of it is causing anxiety or whether retirement is causing a loss of self esteem in either the patient or partner, with concomitant effects on sexual performance. Has the menopause or a hysterectomy changed the way a woman perceives herself? Does she feel less feminine or attractive to her partner or has her sex drive increased with freedom from child rearing, causing disparity between the couple's sexual desires and needs?

These aspects may need very tactful questioning to elicit and require sensitivity on the part of the doctor.

Medical and recreational drugs

Many drugs, especially hypotensives, and the quantity and frequency of alcohol and nicotine intake, can have a profound effect on sexual performance, as can many so called "cold cures" and over the counter hypnotics that contain anticholinergics such as diphenhydramine.

Equally, lack of hormone replacement therapy can cause a major problem in a menopausal woman's sexual relationship, with vaginal atrophy and dryness leading to pain during sexual intercourse, which only direct questioning elicits. This aspect

may not be volunteered by, or even be apparent to, her partner and is a good reason to try to listen to the couple together.

Cannabis can cause an initial euphoria, improving sexual confidence, but, like alcohol, it can greatly diminish ability. Other drugs, including the so called "hard" drugs, have a deleterious long term effect.

Agreeing a management plan

The final part of history taking is for the doctor to decide what is to be done next. A management plan should then be discussed and agreed with the patient. At this point they should decide whether the patient's partner should be invited for a joint meeting if he or she has not been present. In this way, the patient will feel that a partnership exists with the doctor, and treatment is much more likely to succeed.

The picture of placement of seats is reproduced with the subjects' permission. The pictures of defensive body posture and postural echo are reproduced with permission of Mike Wyndham. The picture of extensive penile warts is reproduced with the permission of Dr Colm O'Mahoney and the X ray of an arthritic hip joint, by CRNI is reproduced with permission of Science Photo Library. The chart of commonly prescribed drugs, with an update by Dr Michael Crowe, is reproduced with the permission of Dr Clive Glass.

Commonly prescribed drugs associated with sexual dysfunction (list not fully comprehensive)

Drug	Erectile dysfunction	Loss of desire	Ejaculatory disorder	Orgasmic disorder	Priapism
Anticonvulsants					
Carbamazepine	✓		Also gynaecomastia	✓	
Phenytoin	✓	✓			
Primidone	✓	✓			
Valproate	✓	✓			
Antidepressants*					
Tricyclics					
Amitriptyline	✓	✓	✓	✓	
Amoxapine	✓	✓	✓		
Clomipramine	✓	✓	✓	✓	
Imipramine	✓	✓	✓	✓	
Maprotiline	✓	✓			
Nortriptyline	✓	✓			
Trimipramine	✓	✓	✓	✓	
Monoamine oxidase inhibitors					
Phenelzine	✓	✓	✓	✓	
Selective serotonin reuptake inhibitors					
Fluoxetine	✓		✓		
Fluovoxamine	✓		✓		
Paroxetine	✓		✓		
Sertraline	✓		✓		
Venlafaxine	✓	✓			
Lithium		✓			
Antipsychotics					
Chlorpromazine	✓	✓	✓		✓
Fluphenazine	✓	✓	✓		
Haloperidol	✓		✓		
Amisulpride	✓	✓			
Risperidone	✓	✓			
Zotepine	✓	✓			
Benzodiazepines	✓	✓	✓	✓	
Antihypertensives					
Atenolol	✓				
Bisprolol	✓	✓	✓	✓	
Carvedilol	✓	✓	✓	✓	
Clonidine	✓		✓	✓	
Enalapril	✓				
Felodipine					
Guanethidine	✓	✓	✓		
Hydralazine	✓				✓
Labetalol	✓	✓	✓		✓

Drug	Erectile dysfunction	Loss of desire	Ejaculatory disorder	Orgasmic disorder	Priapism
Lisinopril	✓				
Methyldopa	✓	✓	✓	✓	
Metoprolol	✓	✓			
Pindolol	✓	✓	✓	✓	
Prazosin	✓				✓
Propranolol	✓	✓	✓	✓	
Quinapril	✓				
Ramipril		✓			
Reserpine	✓	✓	✓		
Terazosin					✓
Timolol	✓	✓			
Verapamil	✓				
Lipid regulators					
Bezafibrate	✓				
Fenofibrate	✓				
Gemfibrozil	✓				
H₂ antagonists					
Cimetidine	✓				
Famotidine	✓				
Nizatidine	✓				
Ranitidine	✓				
Diuretics					
Amiloride	✓	✓			
Chlorthalidone	✓	✓			
Indapamide	✓	✓			
Spironolactone	✓	✓			
Thiazides	✓				
Antiemetics					
Metoclopramide	✓	✓			
Non-steroidal anti-inflammatory drugs					
Naproxen	✓		✓		
Anticholinergics					
Atropine	✓				
Diphenhydramine	✓	✓	✓	✓	
Hydroxyzine	✓	✓			
Propantheline	✓				
Scopolamine	✓				
Antispasmodics					
Baclofen	✓		✓		
Hypnotics		✓			
Barbiturates	✓	✓	✓		

*The following antidepressants have little or no sexual side effects: mitrazapine, trazodone, reboxetine, moclobemide, and nefazodone (only available on a named patient basis). Clozapine seems to be without sexual side effects.

5 Examination of patients with sexual problems

John Dean

Examination of a patient with sexual problems involves standard procedures, with which most doctors already will be very familiar. As the focus of the examination is to elicit physical signs relevant to sexual function, however, it can take on a different and more threatening significance for the patient than if performed as part of the assessment of a non-sexual gynaecological or urological problem. The symbolic value of the examination to the patient (and possibly their partner) may well introduce difficulties not experienced in other situations.

Patients may anticipate the examination with dread and profound embarrassment or, conversely, may see it as a potential source of reassurance and relief. Doctors must be aware of the many popular myths about sex and that their patients often may hold quite idiosyncratic beliefs and fears, which will also need to be addressed.

At the outset, the doctor should explain how the examination, which is essential in all patients with a suspected physical problem, might help them and tell them precisely what it entails. An unusual history, odd behaviour by either partner during assessment, inconsistent findings on examination, or unexplained bruising or trauma may alert you to an abusive relationship. Any suspicions should not be ignored, but great care and sensitivity are needed to address this issue.

Requirements for examination

- Privacy, warmth, and an unhurried approach are essential
- A third of women and a fifth of men prefer to be examined by a doctor of their own sex
- Carefully consider cultural mores
- To offer patients a chaperone is prudent for reassurance, as well as medicolegal reasons
- Assess holistically and exclude other diseases that may have a bearing on the sexual problem, such as diabetes, hypertension, and depression

Patient preferences in examination

Physical examination of a patient with a sexual problem should only be done if useful additional information is likely. Some will find examination of the genitalia or breasts deeply embarrassing. Success will depend on their cooperation and confidence in you, and often it is better to defer examination to a later date if the patient is particularly tense and anxious.

Explain why the examination is necessary, what it will involve, and why they may have any discomfort. Make sure you have their permission to do the examination and be prepared to stop it if they ask.

A substantial minority of patients, men and women, prefer to be examined by a doctor of their own sex, so offer them this choice. Remember that allegations of indecent assault have been made even when the examining doctor was of the same sex. Offer a chaperone, but if the offer is declined, record the fact. If a chaperone is present, make a note and record the chaperone's identity.

Cultural differences must also be considered. Many Muslim, Hindu, and Sikh women have a strict sexual morality. Girls are brought up to be shy and modest and submitting to a vaginal examination may be regarded with abhorrence, even as a matter of life and death. Remember that our own sexual mores are not accepted universally. To explore these issues with the patient

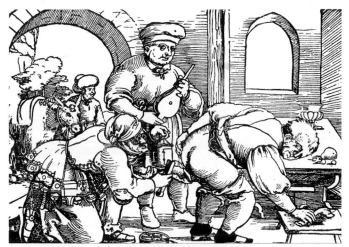

To explain at the outset precisely what an examination entails is important. (*Mercury treatment for venereal disease*, circa 1500)

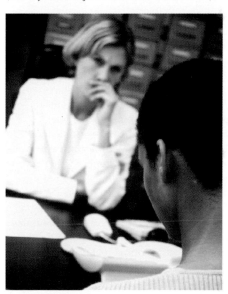

Before patients from ethnic minorities are examined, cultural differences in sexual mores should be considered

Cross cultural issues in taking a history

When a history is taken for patients from cross cultural backgrounds be aware of:
- The patients' own culture, race and ethnicity and how they may impact on the consultation, particularly if you are white and the patients are not
- Your feelings—positive and negative—towards patients from other cultures. Try to gain awareness of your own internalised racism
- Trying to avoid colour blindness and to treat everyone the same. The cultural upbringing of patients from minority groups may mean they have a very different world view from your own. Race, class, education, and socioeconomic factors, as well as those of religion and language, are involved
- A non-judgmental attitude and respect towards patients is needed, especially if the patients hold very different values from your own
- Whether you are able to understand different religious, social, and cultural issues, particularly other cultures' attitudes to the opposite sex
- Your ability to deal with shame or embarrassment, or both, on the part of you or the patient, especially when intimate sexual details need to be discussed
- That the use of language may be very different and that you need to clarify what the patient really means: for example, if an African client talks about discharge, he may be referring to ejaculation

before proceeding with an examination is both wise and a kindness.

General examination

A holistic assessment is important and the doctor should not neglect evidence of concomitant disease that may be a contributory factor to the sexual problem. Cardiovascular, respiratory, or neurological disease may, directly or indirectly, cause sexual problems. Musculoskeletal disorders may lead to sexual problems through chronic pain or immobility. Observe patients' general mobility, spinal mobility, and movement of the hips and knees. A patient's affect may suggest depression, anxiety, or other mental health problems.

Examination of both men and women should include the blood pressure and fasting blood glucose. Both hypertension and its treatments are associated strongly with a range of sexual problems, as is diabetes. Urine testing with a reagent strip is not a reliable test for diabetes and should only be used if phlebotomy is impractical.

Examination of male patients

General

Appearance—Observation of general appearance is important and may reveal signs of androgen deficiency or other endocrine abnormalities. The distribution of facial and body hair and the presence of gynaecomastia should be noted. Many men with androgen deficiency have normal body hair and beard growth. Check blood pressure and radial pulse and palpate the peripheral pulses in men with erectile dysfunction. Evidence of arterial disease, such as absence of foot pulses, suggests an erection problem might be caused by arterial insufficiency.

Nervous system—A detailed examination of the central nervous system is very rarely necessary, but assess the lumbosacral nervous system if the indications are present. A dual innervation of the male reproductive system exists—from the sacral roots (S2-4) through the pudendal and pelvic nerves with predominantly somatic and parasympathetic fibres and from the thoraco-lumbar roots (T11-L2) through the hypogastric, sympathetic, and pelvic nerves. Tactile (dorsal column) and pinprick (spinothalamic tract) sensation in the perineal and lower limb dermatomes should be assessed. The condition of the perineal reflexes may provide evidence of spinal cord dysfunction.

Abdomen—Check for abdominal surgery or intra-abdominal pathology such as an aortic aneurysm and palpable bladder or kidneys. Hernias may also cause pain and sexual problems.

Reflex tests

Reflex	Test
Perianal reflexes	The muscular contractions provoked in these reflexes can usually be seen or palpated
Bulbocavernosus reflex (S2 and S3)	Firmly squeezing the glans penis provokes a contraction of the bulbocavernosus muscle located between the scrotum and anal sphincter
Bulbo-anal reflex (S3 and S4)	Firm squeezing of the glans penis provokes a contraction of the anal sphincter
Anal reflex (S4 and S5)	Stroking or scratching of the skin next to the anus provokes contraction of the anal sphincter

Genital

The appearance of the external genitalia and any apparent developmental anomalies should be noted.

Penis—The size of the flaccid penis is variable, with an unstretched length of between 5-9 cm and a stretched length of

General examination

- Look for evidence of endocrine disease
- Measure blood pressure and take a fasting blood sample for glucose estimation
- Check the cardiovascular and central nervous systems
- Examine the abdomen
- Check the external genitalia and, in men, the anus and prostate

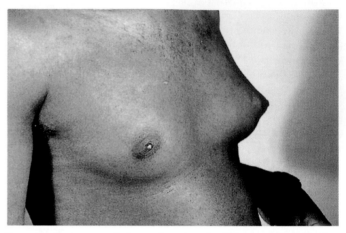

Presence of gynaecomastia in a male patient should be noted. This usually settles spontaneously but, rarely, may be severe enough to warrant breast reduction

Investigations for male sexual dysfunction

In patients with erectile dysfunction
- Urine analysis for glucose or a blood sugar test to exclude diabetes

In patients with loss of sex drive
- Fasting blood glucose
- Testosterone (sample taken at 9 am)
- Sex hormone binding globulin
- Serum albumen
- Free androgen index (calculated from the above)
- Luteinising hormone
- Prolactin
- Luteinising hormone and testosterone have a negative feedback relation similar to that of thyroid stimulating hormone and thyroxine. This can be useful in distinguishing hypogonadism and pituitary disorders as causes of testosterone deficiency
- Prostate specific antigen and other investigations are needed only when coexisting disease is suspected

12 cm. It may seem smaller in obese men, being buried in the pubic fat. The presence of any firm plaques of Peyronie's disease should be assessed. The foreskin, if present, should be retracted, and any pain, restriction, or scarring noted. The position of the urethral orifice should be confirmed, and the presence of genital warts or other infective problems noted.

Testes—The testes should feel smooth and symmetrical. The epididymes can be palpated and, again, should be symmetrical and uniform. The vasa should be palpable as firm whipcords without swellings. A varicocele sometimes can be felt as a swelling above the testicle, more commonly on the left side, and often is seen better in the standing position. They are often cited as a cause of fertility problems or pain, but evidence is inconclusive. No reliable relationship exists between testicular size and androgen levels, although athletes who abuse steroids may have smaller, softer gonads than expected.

Prostate gland—A rectal examination should be performed (and any perianal problems noted) to assess the size and shape of the prostate. The size of the gland can vary, but it should be firm, smooth, and symmetrical, with a uniform consistency (the same firmness as the thenar eminence when the tips of the thumb and forefinger are pressed together), and the median groove should be palpable. It should not be tender to gentle pressure. A gland that feels hard, irregular, or asymmetrical suggests prostatic malignancy. Tenderness often indicates prostatitis, which can be a cause of perineal pain or pain on ejaculation. In either case, further investigation is warranted, and referral to a urological or genitourinary medicine specialist should be considered.

Examination of female patients

General

As in male patients, observation of general appearance is important. Assess the development of secondary sex characteristics and exclude hirsutism and other signs of virilisation. Check the blood pressure, radial pulse, and urine. Examine the abdomen and the reflexes, including a check of the anal reflex if a neurological problem is suspected.

Genital

Inspect the external genitalia for any apparent developmental anomalies. Note the condition of the labia minora, clitoris, urethral orifice, vagina, and anus and whether evidence of warts or other infections is present. Is the vulval skin healthy or is evidence of atrophy and oestrogen deficiency present? Are hymenal remnants or adhesions present? Note evidence of previous childbirth and scarring from perinatal tears or an episiotomy.

Urinary incontinence—If urinary incontinence related to sexual activity is a problem, examination of a patient with a full bladder is essential. Stress incontinence and detrusor instability may be the culprit; the latter sometimes is associated with voiding at orgasm. With the patient in the left lateral position, ask her to cough vigorously while you observe the urethral orifice: a jet of urine suggests stress incontinence. If incontinence is a problem, referral for urodynamic assessment by a urologist or gynaecologist is prudent.

Speculum examination should be performed, and any pain or vaginal discharge during the procedure should be noted. The appearance of the vagina and cervix should be assessed, and, if appropriate, bacterial and chlamydial swabs may be taken from the vagina and endocervical canal. Exclusion of chlamydiasis especially is important in women who complain of dyspareunia. A holistic assessment is important and evidence of concomitant disease that may be a contributory factor to the sexual problem should not be neglected. Cardiovascular, respiratory, or

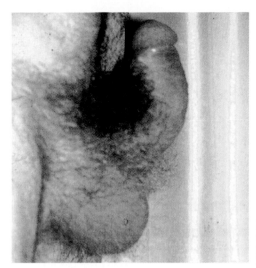

Peyronie's deformity caused by the presence of a dorsal plaque in the penis

---

Rectal examination

Look for anal warts, haemorrhoids, sinus, or fissure

The prostate
- Should be smooth and symmetrical with the firmness of a tensed thenar eminence
- May be tender but should not be painful
- Hardness, irregularity, or asymmetry suggests malignancy and needs urgent referral

---

Examination of a female patient
- Examination is necessary only when a physical problem is suspected and may not always be appropriate
- Note the general appearance
- Check secondary sexual characteristics, as well as pulse, blood pressure, and urine
- Examine cardiovascular system, central nervous system, abdomen, and external genitalia
- To assess stress incontinence, examine patient with a full bladder and ask her to cough
- Digital and speculum examination of the vagina should be made carefully
- Rectal examination rarely is necessary

Investigations for female sexual dysfunction
- Endocrine investigation has a limited role but is necessary in women with menstrual irregularity or other symptoms of oestrogen deficiency
- If ovarian failure with oestrogen deficiency is suspected, check estradiol (day 6 if premenopausal), follicle stimulating hormone and luteinising hormone. Estradiol may be unreliable if the woman is taking synthetic or equine oestrogens
- Prolactin to exclude a pituitary prolactinoma
- Thyroxine—as in men, hyperthyroidism and hypothyroidism can cause dysfunction in sexual drive and arousal
- If loss of sexual desire is an important feature, check thyroid function and prolactin, plus sex hormone binding globulin and albumen to calculate the free testosterone level
- Other investigations are necessary only when coexisting disease is suspected

neurological disease directly or indirectly may cause sexual problems. Musculoskeletal disorders may lead to sexual problems through chronic pain or immobility. Observe patients' general mobility, spinal mobility, and movement of the hips and knees. A patient's manner may suggest depression, anxiety, or other mental health problems.

Gentle digital examination of the vagina helps to identify tenderness and muscle spasm. If tolerated, a bimanual examination should be performed to assess the condition of the cervix, uterus, and adnexa. Particularly note any tenderness, thickening, or swellings: their presence often will need referral for further assessment by a gynaecologist. The position of the uterus, either anteverted or retroverted, can be noted, but this rarely is of relevance as a cause of sexual problems. Beware of commenting on the position of the uterus to your patient unless you are prepared to address the matter fully.

Rectal examination in a woman is rarely necessary unless an anal or rectal problem is suspected. Do look at the perianal skin, however, for evidence of scarring, warts, or infection.

Conclusion

When the examination of the patient has been concluded, you must give the patient as clear an explanation of the findings as possible. The findings often are entirely normal, and this reassurance can be very important as a first step in a patient's recovery of their sexual wellbeing.

The picture of treatment of venereal disease is reproduced with permission of Mary Evans Picture Library. The picture of gynaecomastia is reproduced with permission of the Wellcome Photo Library. The photographs of the speculum (Simon Fraser) and the consultation (BSIP, LA, Filin Herrera) are with permission of the Science Photo Library. The photograph of perianal warts is courtesy of Dr Colm O'Mahoney.

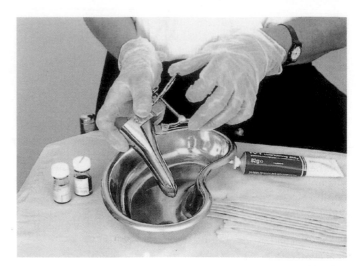
Duck bill speculum used to hold open the vagina during examination and for swabs to be taken

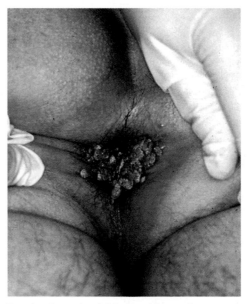
Examine the perianal skin for evidence of warts

6 Female sexual problems I: loss of desire—what about the fun?

Josie Butcher

Loss of desire for sexual activity is the most common presenting female sexual dysfunction and often is the hardest to treat. Whether such loss of sexual desire should be seen as abnormal or simply a variation of normal has long been debated. Much literature that considers sexuality for women from various angles is available on female loss of desire. The American Psychiatric Association's *Diagnostic and Statistical Manual of Mental Disorders* (DSM-IV-TR), fourth edition, text revision gives an accepted working classification of psychosexual dysfunction. It classifies desire problems as hypoactive sexual desire disorder and sexual aversion disorder. Hypoactive sexual desire disorder is defined as a deficiency or absence of sexual fantasy or desire for sexual activity, and must cause personal distress or interpersonal difficulty, or both.

An adaptation of Masters and Johnson's original "human sexual response curve" helps us to consider loss of desire in the context of the normal sexual response. This representation describes the sequence of physiological events that takes place and measures increasing sexual pleasure against time. Sexual desire can be followed by arousal, orgasm, and finally resolution or can be consequent on engaging in sexual stimuli that produces arousal. Remember, however, that the physiologies of the different phases are separate entities and therefore are not dependent on each other. Women with loss of desire can have good sexual function. In essence, they are not likely to initiate sexual contact and have little motivation to seek sexual stimuli.

Is desire a thought or a feeling? The answer is not clear, and, certainly early in loving relationships, genital arousal often closely follows any sexual thought. The initial sexual thought facilitates the arousal mechanism through neurological pathways. This thought could be anticipation of the evening ahead or a memory of a previous sexual encounter. Many women who do not have spontaneous desire for sexual activity can operate quite well sexually once engaged in the sexual encounter and enjoy sexual stimuli such as touch around the clitoris and genital area, which facilitates neurological pathways, producing good arousal, often development of sexual desire, and progression to orgasm.

Two models are useful to consider. In Riley's model, sexual drive is described as the need for sexual activity, possibly recognised by the presence of spontaneous sexual thoughts, with sexual desire being the focus of sexual drive.[1] The Basson model looks at engaging in sexual stimuli from a position of sexual neutrality—the resultant arousal leads to development of desire.[2]

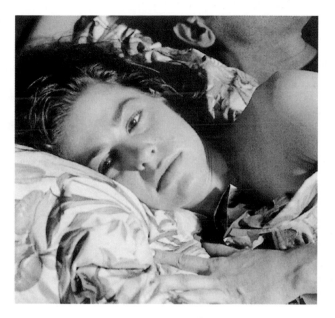

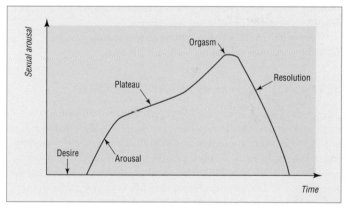

The normal female sexual response. Adapted from Masters WH, Johnson VE. *Human sexual response*. Boston, MA: Little, Brown, 1966

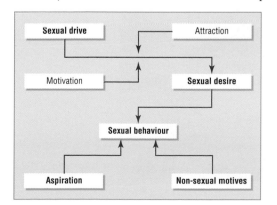

Model of sexual response. (Adapted from Riley (1997)[1])

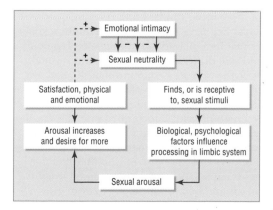

Model of sexual responding. (Adapted from Basson (2002)[2])

21

Causes of loss of sexual desire

Much research into sexual desire is being undertaken, but it is still poorly understood. We know that certain medical conditions affect it, such as depression, stress, and fatigue.

Organic causes

Research strongly suggests that androgens have a part to play in women's sexual desire, although much smaller amounts are needed than in men. In women, testosterone production is split evenly between the ovaries and adrenal gland, and androgen deficiency syndrome should be considered after hysterectomy and bilateral salpingo-oophorectomy and after chemotherapy for cancer. Treatment with testosterone can improve loss of desire in some cases.

The effect of changing hormone patterns at different life stages is poorly understood, but it is well known that loss of desire is more common with premenstrual tension, postnatally, and around the menopause. Hyperprolactinaemia of any aetiology can have a direct effect on reduction of sexual drive or desire, and many drugs, such as antiepileptic drugs, can cause loss of desire.

Any health problem or drug history (prescribed or recreational) that might affect sexual anatomy, the vascular system, the neurological system, and the endocrine system must be considered. Indirect causes are conditions that can cause dyspareunia, chronic pain, fatigue, and malaise and that interfere with the vascular and neurological pathways. A careful history therefore is important. As the physiology of sexual drive and desire becomes more understood, much excitement surrounds the understanding of the neurotransmitters involved and the potential for medical treatments.

We must remember that loss of desire simply can be secondary to poor sexual arousal and orgasm.

Sense of self as a sexual person

Often it is difficult to disentangle organic possibilities from psychogenic variables that occur in women at different life stages and the effect that these may have on how women see sexuality fitting into their lives. To consider these points and not allow ourselves to be dragged into the medical model is important. We should look at the importance of the different roles that women have in their lives and how they prioritise them.

Many women have several roles—the professional or worker, housewife, mother, daughter, friend, and lover. Often it seems that the last role fades away as the demands of other roles increase. When a woman meets her first serious partner, she usually has fewer of these, but in her later years, she will have more roles with which to contend.

Observation of these issues can be quite revealing, and it is useful to ask a woman her views on her learning about sexuality and the influences that have played a part in its development. Sexual learning and role prioritisation often are intertwined. An example of this is the woman who found that she had lost sexual desire after the birth of her first child. Discussion showed that she had, not unnaturally, made the responsibility of being a mother a high priority, but coupled with this was the clear message that she had received when learning about her sexuality, that "mothers are not sexual beings."

For women to understand the sense of who they feel they are as sexual beings is important, and it gives women insight into their sexual needs and behaviour. An easy way to give structure to this is to undertake a "timetable of life." Both partners in the relationship are asked to fill in a timetable that

Possible causes of hyperprolactinaemia
- Pituitary tumours
- Hypothyroidism
- Cirrhosis
- Stress
- Hypothalamic diseases
- Hepatic disease
- Breast surgery
- Drug treatments

Illnesses that may result in loss of sexual desire
- Gynaecological disorders causing pain on sexual intercourse
- Obstetric disorders causing pain on sexual intercourse
- Urological disorders causing pain on sexual intercourse
- Alcohol and substance misuse
- Stress and chronic anxiety
- Endocrine disorders
- Neurological disorders
- Psychiatric disorders
- Depression
- Fatigue

Drugs that can affect women's sexual function
- Antiandrogens
  Cyproterone
  Gonadotrophin releasing hormone analogues
- Antioestrogens and other hormones
  Tamoxifen
- Contraceptive drugs
- Cytotoxic drugs
- Psychoactive drugs
  Sedatives
  Narcotics
  Antidepressants
  Neuroleptics
  Stimulants

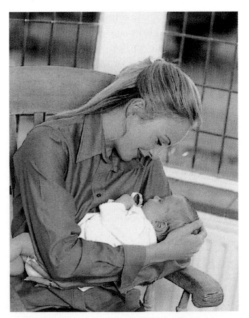

As a woman takes on the roles of mother and housewife, the importance of the role of lover may diminish

shows a typical week. They then are asked to look at the week in terms of time spent in different categories: family time (with children and partners), work time (at work and work in the house), extended family time (with parents and relations), social time, personal time, and relationship time (time spent together alone, as a couple). This last category is, of course, the time when sexual activity is more likely to be realised successfully.

The roles women take on in life and how they prioritise them are not just about the practicalities of who does what, but more the responsibilities of roles that women feel. A timetable almost inevitably shows little priority given to relationship time and personal time.

A repeat of this exercise with timetables for different times in a woman's life to allow comparison of the timetable during courtship, when sexual desire was probably good, and the timetable for a time when sexual desire was low is useful. Discussion around changes in life's priorities and the impact of these on sexual activity usually follows. Exploration of areas such as partner attraction, aspirations and expectations of relationships, intimacy, and commitment allows patients to gain insight.

Many misunderstandings and myths can be acquired during learning about sexuality: such as that a man is always ready and able to have sex, that sex is natural and spontaneous, and that sex equals intercourse. Sexual myths are held by women as well as men.

Treatment options

An integrated approach to medical and psychological treatments is optimal. Any medical elements of the problem, if present, must be treated to achieve a positive outcome. In secondary loss of desire for sexual activity, a psychogenic aspect often remains after the medical elements have been treated.

In today's society, acknowledgement that understanding of the female sexual system as a whole is improved is important. Research is now centred around female sexual physiology, and much interest has been placed on possible options for drug treatment. We still have much to learn about the complexity of female sexual desire, but, so far, research into this area has not given many answers.

In many studies, this complexity is shown. Although physiological improvement in arousal can be measured after drug treatment, statistically significant changes in function, drive, and satisfaction still are not proven.

Some studies have looked at different aspects of sexual desire and have expressed the idea of it as an adaptive function to boost attachment and develop bonding. Other studies have looked at cycles based on intimacy.

The mainstays of treatment are still centred around cognitive, behavioural, and psychodynamic approaches.

One of the most difficult areas to approach and deal with is loss of attraction for the partner, which can lead to serious difficulties and consequences. When loss of sexual desire is present, work with people as couples allows both partners' understanding of the problem (which is examined by means of some of the techniques described above). As partners begin to realise that they can no longer assume that they know how their partner feels, or should feel, the differences in sexuality and sexual needs can be explored. We expect our partners to feel the same way as we feel and to know when we feel sexual. We expect them to be able to provide for our needs sexually without necessarily discussing them.

Possible sources for sexual learning include parental values, religious teaching, cultural mores, and life events

---

Myths about sex

1 Men are very comfortable about sex
2 In general, a man should not be seen to express certain emotions
3 All physical contact must lead to sex
4 A man wants and is always ready for sex
5 In sex, as elsewhere, it is performance that counts
6 A hard penis is essential for a satisfying sexual experience
7 If you can't get a hard penis, there is a pill that will take care of it
8 Sex equals intercourse
9 Good sex must follow a linear progression of increasing excitement and terminate in orgasm
10 Sex should be natural and spontaneous
11 On the whole, the man must take charge of and orchestrate sex
12 We no longer believe the above myths

*Adapted from Zilbergeld B. *The new male sexuality*, Revised edn. London: Bantam, 1999

Diagnostic checklist for women's loss of sexual desire

- Physical illness
- Integrity of anatomy
- Integrity of vascular system
- Integrity of neurological system
- Integrity of endocrine system
- Drugs and treatments
- Psychological characteristics
- Relationship issues
- Life changes
- Sexual history
- Sexual knowledge
- Attraction to partner

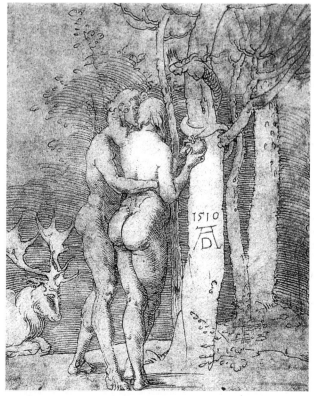

We expect our partners to feel the same way as we feel and to know when we feel sexual. *Callpygous Eve and Adoring Adam* (1510) by Albrecht Dürer

Much success has been gained by helping women to understand their sense of self. This process often is empowering; it allows women to break away from the concept of being dysfunctional and allows desire to re-establish itself. It is important to remember that sexual drive, desire, behaviour, and satisfaction are complex and not easily equated to a purely medical model.

> **Frigidity does not feature in this discussion or in any classification of female sexual dysfunction. The term is more a reflection of women's feelings about themselves or men's feelings about women. When a woman describes herself as frigid, she really is describing how she feels about herself as a sexual being, and often this is a comparison with her or others' expectations of how she should feel and be. Frigidity is not a medical term, and it no longer should be used**

1 Riley A. Psychosexual disorders: problems of the sexual response cycle. *Diplomate* 1997;4:270-5
2 Basson R. Female sexual dysfunction—the new models. *Br J Diab Vasc Dis* 2002;2:267-70

Further reading
- Bancroft J. *Human sexuality and its problems*. Edinburgh: Churchill Livingstone, 1998
- Kaplan HS. *The sexual desire disorders*. New York: Brunner Mazel, 1995
- Crowe M, Ridley J. *Therapy with couples*. Oxford: Blackwell Science, 1990 (reprinted 1996)
- Masters WH, Johnson VE, Kolodny RC. *Human sexuality*. New York: Harper Collins, 1995
- Leiblum SR, Rosen RC. *Principles and practices of sex therapy*. London: Guildford Press, 2000

7 Female sexual problems II: sexual pain and orgasmic disorders

Josie Butcher

Dyspareunia and vaginismus are two common and extremely frustrating sexual dysfunctions for women. The American Psychiatric Association's *Diagnostic and Statistical Manual of Mental Disorders*, fourth edition, text revision (DSM-IV-TR), lists them as two separate disorders in the subcategory of sexual dysfunctions. The International Consensus Development Conference, however, add to this category non-coital sexual pain disorder—an important recognition that sexual pain not always is related to sexual intercourse or play.[1]

Dyspareunia

Dyspareunia is defined as a recurrent and persistent genital pain associated with sexual activity. It is classified as primary, when pain has always occurred during sexual activity, or secondary, when it occurs after a period of pain free lovemaking. The term is used usually to describe pain on penetration, but it can occur during genital stimulation. Dyspareunia is described best according to the site of pain.

Traditionally, superficial dyspareunia (at or around the vaginal entrance) was thought likely to have a psychogenic origin, whereas deep dyspareunia was likely to have an organic cause. These explanations are no longer considered helpful. It is important to try to identify the history of the pain, its site, type, severity, onset, duration, and any other associated factors. Any physical abnormalities must be looked for, and their effects on the sexual relationship should be discussed. Remember that physical signs are not always visible, and vulval histology is sometimes needed, although it is not always helpful. To suggest that dyspareunia is simply psychological is never enough; it should be looked at medically before any psychological components are considered.

Repeated sexual pain can set up a cycle of pain, however, in which fear of the pain leads to avoidance of the sexual activity that produces it, which in turn leads to lack of arousal, failure to achieve orgasm, and loss of sexual desire. This can progress to total avoidance of sexual activity and difficulties in a woman's relationship with her partner.

Superficial vulval pain

Superficial vulval pain is common and has many causes. Identification of the cause is difficult, however, and patients often see treatments as frustrating and inadequate. There is a great risk of a patient focusing on the discomfort and repeatedly trying to find answers. She may consider herself misunderstood, and her doctor may become frustrated through failure to find a cure. Although patients are anxious and may be introspective about their symptoms, they seem psychologically "healthy."

Vulval pain can be relapsing and remitting. Experiences of burning, itching, and stinging—with patients describing feeling "inflamed"—are common, and any area of the perineum may be affected. Pain may be felt not only on sexual stimulation but can be present all the time and triggered by non-sexual activities such as walking. The main physical causes are vulvitis, vulvovaginitis, vulvar vestibulitis, vulvodynia, genital herpes,

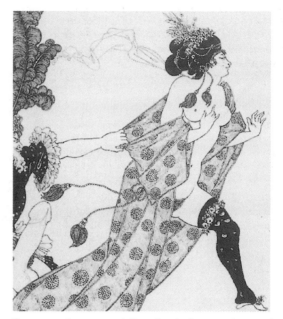

One reason for a woman's fear of vaginal penetration may be a belief that her vagina is too small. (*Cineasias entreating Myrrhina to coition*, 1896, by Aubrey Beardsley)

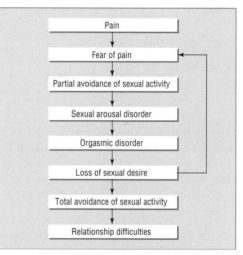

Cycle of sexual pain and avoidance of sexual activity

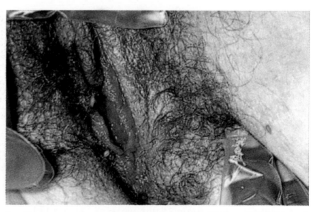

Small sores on vulva caused by herpes simplex II virus. Genital herpes is a major cause of superficial dyspareunia

urethritis, and atrophic vulvitis, as well as inadequate lubrication and topical irritants such as spermicides or latex.

Vaginal pain

To discuss vaginal pain without mention of vaginismus, which in the DSM-IV-TR classification is defined separately, would be inappropriate. The themes for the two, however, are common and intertwining. Pain is mainly experienced at the entrance to the vagina because sensory nerve endings are present only in the lower third. Common causes are lack of lubrication, vaginal infection, irritants (such as spermicides and latex), urethral problems, gynaecological and obstetric interventions (such as episiotomy), radiotherapy (such as radiation vaginitis), and sexual trauma.

Deep dyspareunia

Deep dyspareunia, often described as pain that results from pelvic thrusting during sexual intercourse, also is common and has many causes. Major physical causes include pelvic inflammatory disease; gynaecological, pelvic, or abdominal surgery; postoperative adhesions; endometriosis; genital or pelvic tumours (including fibroids); irritable bowel syndrome; urinary tract infections; and ovarian cysts. Two common causes include lack of arousal and position, with deep thrusting by the woman's partner hitting an ovary (equivalent to hitting or squeezing a man's testicle).

Treatment

When considering treatments for dyspareunia, all physical causes should be treated as far as possible. Cognitive behavioural programmes can be useful, however; they are similar to the approach used for vaginismus (see below). Many women, once they understand their sexual problem, can adapt and achieve good quality sexual activity leading to penetration, even though they have a painful physical condition. Successful treatment largely results from the patient feeling that she owns her vagina and controls her sexual activity.

Vaginismus

Vaginismus is defined as a conditioned response that results from the association of sexual activity with pain and fear. It is a severe problem for many women, who may experience not only extreme physical pain on attempted penetration but also severe psychological pain. It consists of a phobia of penetration of the vagina and involuntary spasm of the pubococcygeal and associated muscles that surround the lower third of the vagina.

Primary vaginismus is diagnosed when a woman has never experienced vaginal penetration, and secondary vaginismus is diagnosed when a woman has had vaginal penetration without a problem in the past.

The severity of the symptoms can lead to a general sexual inhibition with avoidance of any sexual touching, and in most severe cases to avoidance of any affectionate touching. The spasm can occur not only on attempted penetration but on anticipated penetration or foreplay. At the other end of the spectrum, some women are sexually responsive and have good quality sexual experiences, with imaginative "foreplay" continuing to orgasm but avoiding penetration.

Attempted penetration leads to pain, fear, humiliation, and frustration, and often results in feelings of inadequacy and abandonment. The discomfort from repeated attempts at penetration or speculum examination can produce a tightening of muscles in the pelvis, thighs, abdomen, and legs. As well as unsuccessful intercourse, women will have experienced failed gynaecological examinations and difficulty using tampons, and

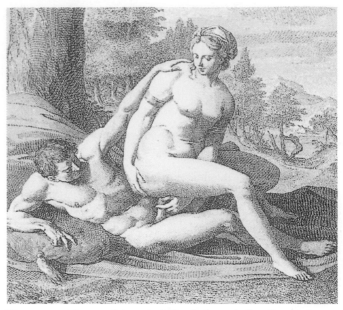

When women take complete control of vaginal penetration, they can learn to overcome their fear of sexual activity. (*Angelique et Medor* from *Aretiono or The Loves of the Gods*, circa 1602, by Agostino Caracci)

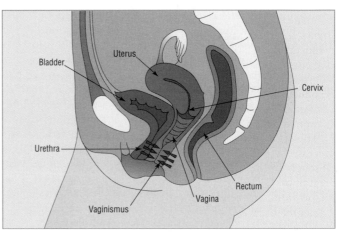

Diagram of vaginismus. (Redrawn from Masters WH, Johnson VE, Kolodny RC. *Human sexuality*. New York: Harper Collins, 1995)

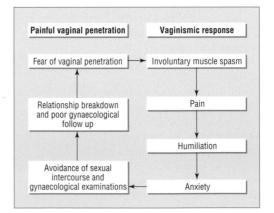

Cycle of vaginismus

will have defaulted from attendance for cytology (of cervical smears), all of which are almost impossible.

Causes

The immediate cause of vaginismus, whether primary or secondary, is involuntary muscle spasm. The reason that some women develop vaginismus and others do not is uncertain. The initial response may be secondary to any type of vaginal pain, including all causes of dyspareunia. Experience of physical or sexual abuse can induce phobia of vaginal penetration, as can frightening medical procedures experienced during childhood, painful first sexual intercourse, problems with a relationship, and fear of pregnancy.

Masters and Johnson suggested that important factors may include religious orthodoxy, poor sexual education, sexual inhibition, sexual abuse, rape, and anger in relationships. Other suggested factors include fear of intimacy, pregnancy, or aggression and belief that the vagina is too small. There is a suggestion that psychological conflict can be implicated; in this, a woman indirectly expresses anger towards her partner by closing off her vagina to him.

Treatment

Cognitive behavioural treatment programmes for vaginismus comprise work to address the phobia coupled with a programme of relaxation, with specific exercises for relaxing the muscles and a systematic desensitisation of the vagina. As previously stated, it is helpful to integrate this type of programme into the treatment of dyspareunia of any cause, as it can lead to improved outcomes.

During such a programme, the woman learns to control her vaginal muscle spasm while gently introducing trainers of gradually increasing size into the vagina. Trainers can be fingers or tampons or they can be specifically designed products such as Amielle trainers. Throughout, the woman is in total control, and this gives her great confidence. The programme progresses to a point where she is able to share the introduction of the trainers with her partner. This stage is followed by insertion of the penis into the vagina, again with the woman in control.

The phobic element of the condition also needs to be addressed and is often the most difficult part of the treatment. Although women may dread the prospect of the treatment programme, the success rate is nearly 100% if the woman persists with it. The aim is to achieve a situation where the woman feels that she owns her own vagina and can share it for sexual activity should she wish.

Research in progress

Other possible interventions are under investigation.

Female orgasmic disorder (anorgasmia)

The role of orgasm for women is not well defined. For some, it is extremely important and sought at every sexual encounter. For others, however, it seems less important and sometimes of little relevance; many women can be quite content without it. An important issue is the male partner's understanding of the female orgasm. He often feels that, like him, his partner cannot fully enjoy sexual activity without it, and this can put enormous pressure on the woman to achieve it.

A working definition of anorgasmia would be an involuntary inhibition of the orgasmic reflex. A woman may have a strong sexual desire with good arousal and enjoy the sensation of the penis in the vagina, but she then holds back even though the stimulation should be sufficient for orgasm. These women often have a strong fear of losing control over feelings and behaviour. The fear can be conscious or unconscious, but resolution of the conflict is an important aim of treatment. An example of a situational anorgasmia is a woman who can achieve orgasm by masturbation but not in coupled sexual activity.

Treating vaginismus

1—Sexual education
2—Control of vaginal muscles
3—Self exploration of sexual anatomy
4—Insertion of a trainer under controlled relaxation
5—Sharing of control with partner
6—Insertion of penis, with the woman in control
7—Transfer control of insertion of penis to partner
8—Exploration of phobia

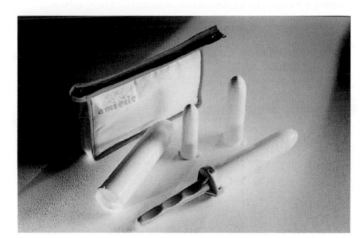

Amielle trainers, which can be used to help overcome fear of vaginal penetration

---

Research in progress

Vulval pain

Vulvodynia
- Use of topical nitroglycerine

Vulvar vestibulitis
- Physical therapies and electromyographic feedback of pelvic floor musculature
- Some studies of surgical treatments have shown good response
- Sensory functions—exploration of the sensory function of the genital area compared with the deltoid area suggests the presence of some generalised systemic hypersensitivity

Vaginismus and dyspareunia
- Rethinking these sexual dysfunctions as pain disorders that interfere with normal sexual functioning
- Use of integrated pain models in treatment programmes (see Cycle of sexual pain at start of chapter)

Psychological and quality of life profiles
These continue to be explored

Classification of anorgasmia

Primary	Orgasm never achieved
Secondary	Orgasm achieved in the past
Absolute	Orgasm impossible in all situations
Situational	Orgasm impossible only in certain situations

Historically, orgasm has been equated with loss of control leading to death and has been described as the "mini-death." Most women who seek help feel that having an orgasm will change their lives dramatically. Education and rational discussion is important in disassociating orgasm from its symbolic qualities.

Treatment

Work with the woman and the couple aims to treat the "holding back"—the fear or phobia of orgasm or losing control. Resolution of conflicts (decreasing inhibitions) combined with increasing stimulation is very successful.

A considerable amount of couple work, during which sexual education, sexual myths, and a greater understanding of a partner's needs can be discussed, is helpful. The question, "Who is this orgasm for?" can be addressed. The idea of difference can be achieved, and the concept of benign variation of sexual need can be accepted.

The picture of genital herpes, by Dr P Marazzi, is reproduced with permission of Science Photo Library

1 Basson R, Berman J, Burnett A et al. Report of the International Consensus Development Conference on female sexual dysfunctions: definitions and classifications. *J Urol* 2000;63:888-93

Treatment of anorgasmia

1—Self exploration
2—Sensate focus
3—Masturbation
4—Use of adjuncts (vibrators)
5—Resolution of unconscious fears of orgasm
6—Distraction
7—Exercises to heighten sexual arousal
8—Transfer to heterosexual situation
9—Orgasm on sexual intercourse

Objectives of treatment

- Heighten sexual arousal so that woman is close to orgasm before penetration
- Enhance awareness of pleasure and vaginal sensation with tactile stimulation in outer third of the vagina
- Maximise clitoral stimulation with active thrusting by woman, woman in superior position, direct clitoral stimulation, use of a vibrator, and use of external clitoral stimulation by woman

Further reading

- Heiman JR, LoPiccolo J. *Becoming orgasmic. A sexual and personal growth programme for women.* London: Piatkus Books, 1999
- Dickson A. *The mirror within.* London: Quartet Books, 2000
- Goodwin AJ, Agronin ME. *A woman's guide to overcome sexual fear and pain.* Oakland: New Harbinger Publications, 1997

8 A woman's sexual life after an operation

Margot Huish, Asun de Marquiegui

Disfiguring and mutilating operations, especially of the face, breasts, genitals, and reproductive organs, often have a deleterious effect on a woman's self image and sexuality. Sociopsychological aspects of body image form a complex pattern of self knowledge and how a person is perceived by others. The invasion of surgery invariably causes temporary or permanent changes that may not be anticipated by women or may emerge only on discharge from hospital.

Partners who adapt poorly to the new circumstances may also find it difficult to continue sexual activity. An existing strong and intimate relationship, however, encourages positive postoperative adjustment.

To deal with psychological and emotional states, such as anxiety, fear, and depression about surgery, is crucial to a woman and her partner. Medical teams should encourage women to discuss their worries, especially sexual anxieties, as problems become more entrenched and more difficult to treat over time. Postoperative surveys of women suggest 28-50% wanted their doctor to address sexual difficulties. Rehabilitation is important in promoting adjustment and acceptance by facilitating the grieving process.

Ileostomy, colostomy, and urostomy

Women who have a stoma as a result of chronic illness, such as irritable bowel disorder, ulcerative colitis, and Crohn's disease, often experience a better psychological and sexual outcome than those who undergo emergency surgery for, say, cancer of the colon. Healthy adaptation to a stoma depends on preoperative and postoperative counselling and understanding by stoma nurses. Patients' greatest fears are loss of control, bad odour, noise, leaking or bursting bags, unsightliness, and their partner's feelings towards them.

Some time may be needed before a couple resumes lovemaking after surgery, particularly if attention is focused on the patient's survival or if complications, such as ill fitting appliances, parastomal sepsis, and skin excoriation, are present. Dyspareunia can be a major problem—not only because of lack of arousal or secondary vaginismus after surgery but because of the amount of scar tissue within the pelvis.

Hip surgery

Total or partial hip replacement is a common operation now, but when a patient can safely resume sex often is not mentioned. Anatomically, internal rotation is dangerous immediately after surgery, because it can lead to dislocation, but, as intercourse usually requires external rotation of the joint and thus dislocation is less likely, sex generally can be resumed when the scar is comfortable.

Heart operations and angina

Although these operations are often done as lifesaving operations with very good outcomes, women must be allowed to discuss their fears about when or if it is safe to restart sexual activity. Intercourse can take place when a woman feels like it, as long as she can walk up two flights of stairs without difficulty— the equivalent cardiac output of orgasm. Angina may limit her activity, although this is unlikely. After a chest operation, the

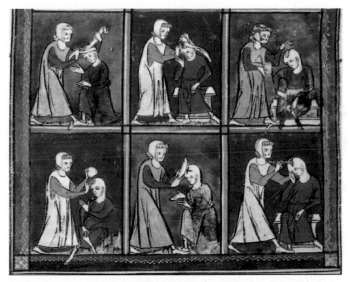
Disfiguring operations, especially of the face and sexual organs, often have a deleterious effect on a woman's self image and sexuality. (Detail from *On surgery* (14th century manuscript) by Rogier de Salerne)

Factors that affect sexual function after an operation
- Disfigurement or mutilation altering the body image
- Previous psychological and emotional states
- Physical pain and hormonal, vascular, or nervous damage
- Existing problems with intimacy and quality of relationship

---

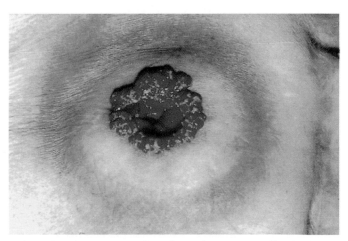
Healthy adaptation to a stoma depends on adequate counselling for the patient and her partner

woman should take the female superior or another comfortable position until discomfort from the chest scar has eased.

Eye operations

Cataract removal places no restrictions on sexual activity, but intercourse should be avoided for two weeks after a retinal detachment. Patients with vitreous haemorrhages need to wait until laser treatment has finished or, if they do not have diabetes, two weeks after bleeding has stopped.

Gynaecological operations

Hysterectomy

The uterus, menstruation, and fertility are seen by many women as fundamental to their femininity. After hysterectomy, women often have great difficulty becoming sexually aroused, particularly when signs of depression are present before the operation and the woman is aged less than 40 years. In some women for whom other treatments have not worked, however, hysterectomy can be a relief from heavy bleeding, pain, and tiredness and allows a freer sexual life. A change of sensation from pins and needles to numbness on the inner aspect of the thighs can occur. If sensation is going to return, it can take up to a year.

Intercourse usually is avoided for six weeks, but this is somewhat arbitrary. Variation of positions, such as lying on the side or rear entry, should be tried to reduce the depth of vaginal penetration, as the vaginal length can be reduced by up to a third after hysterectomy or trachelectomy. Gentle penetration is possible after four weeks, although many women prefer to wait for longer.

Vaginal repairs

These are done mainly for prolapse of the bladder or rectum. Some women complain of postoperative vaginal tightness or dyspareunia because of tender scar tissue. They should be encouraged to restart sexual intercourse when it feels comfortable and to use a water based lubricant such as KY Jelly or Senselle, or an aromatic oil such as peach kernel or sweet almond oil (oils must not be used with barrier contraceptives made from latex rubber, as these can perish and split in less than a minute; polyurethane condoms are not affected).

Incontinence and colloid injections

Sexual expression can be affected badly by incontinence, with fears about odour, leakage, and wetness. If a woman tenses her pubococcygeal muscles and bladder sphincter in order not to dribble urine, the resulting physiological and psychological tension can lead to vaginismus and possibly dyspareunia and interference with sexual arousal and orgasm.

Minor operations

The diagnosis of an abnormal cervical smear can create great anxiety, especially when totally unexpected. A woman must be allowed to express her anxiety and fears about cervical cancer and its effect on her sex life before she is referred for colposcopy. The woman will then find it easier to resume her sexual life after treatment.

Female genital mutilation

This operation is illegal in Britain, but the obstetric and sexual sequelae are seen in clinics in areas with large African and Middle Eastern communities. Recent arrivals may need deinfibulation because they are getting married or are pregnant. Young women brought up in Britain may feel mutilated

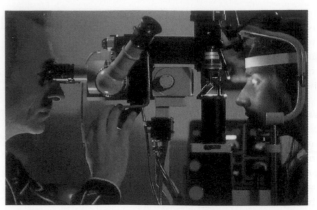

Patients who undergo laser treatment for a detached retina or vitreous haemorrhage should be warned to avoid sexual activity until treatment has finished

A 49 year old housewife of average intelligence came to a family planning clinic eight weeks after undergoing a hysterectomy. She was worried about not having had a period yet and wanted to find out when she could resume sexual intercourse. She had not felt able to ask at the gynaecology clinic because everyone was so busy

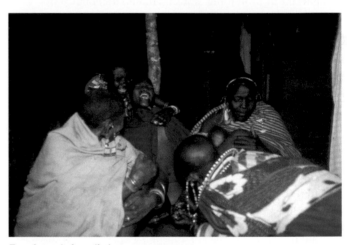

Female genital mutilation

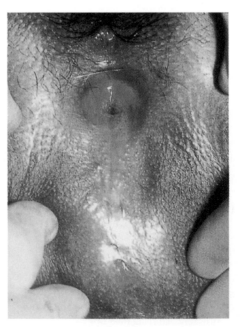

Examination of a woman who had undergone ritual genital mutilation as a child and who now needs deinfibulation to enable her to reproduce

compared with their peers and will need appropriate sexual counselling and occasionally deinfibulation. Problems with non-consummation of marriage are common, often because of vaginismus. Women who have undergone this operation should be examined by doctors comfortable with the treatment of psychosexual problems.

Episiotomies, obstetric tears, and trauma
Episiotomies have been done routinely to prevent tears in the perineum during labour. It is essential that midwives and junior doctors are trained properly and should take great care in the site and length of incision and its repair to protect the perineum. Poor repairs that lead to malposition of the sutures, painful scars, narrowing of the introitus, or even extrusion of pieces of catgut can affect sexual pleasure severely.

As low sexual desire, dyspareunia, and secondary vaginismus are common responses after childbirth, women may benefit from postnatal referral to a therapist to discuss sexual dysfunction. Psychological reasons are varied, but tiredness, especially when breast feeding, and fears of a further pregnancy also can have a negative effect on a sexual relationship. A woman's focus on her body as a mother rather than as a lover can also affect sexual function.

Termination of pregnancy
Some women feel relieved after a termination and the operation has little impact on their psychological wellbeing, but others may feel a deep sense of loss and grief. This causes anxiety, depression, loss of sexual desire, and difficulties within an existing relationship. When this happens, the reasons the termination was wanted need to be explored, and all the emotions of that loss need to be counselled. Intercourse can be resumed when the woman has stopped bleeding after the termination if she feels like it.

Sterilisation
Women older than 30 years who have completed their family, especially those who have had problems with contraception, may find that their sexual activity improves after elimination of the possibility of unwanted pregnancies. They can resume intercourse as soon as they feel physically comfortable after the operation. On the other hand, women coerced for family or other reasons into unwanted sterilisation may retreat sexually.

Operations for infertility
The pressure to perform to a calendar gives rise to many sexual problems for men and women. The low success rate of treatments also increases the feelings of failure, loss, grief, frustration, and depression. Couples need counselling to maintain their sexual intimacy while undergoing medical and surgical interventions and beyond.

Operations for cancer
Operations such as hysterectomy, bilateral oophorectomy, and radical vulvectomy can cause major genital mutilation and often produce difficult psychosexual problems. Women have to deal not only with the fear and anxiety of the diagnosis and treatment but the constant fear of recurrence. They often do not know what to expect sexually after an operation because of lack of communication with their doctors, as well as with their partners.

Partners mainly suffer in silence and find it difficult to make sexual approaches. They fear being seen as selfish or not understanding the physical and emotional pain that the woman is going through if they do, or they may put more pressure on her by assuming that she does want sex. Some partners find that

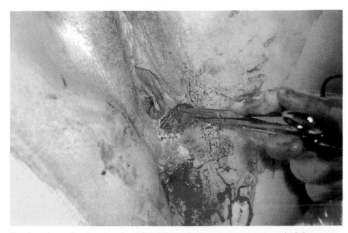

Exploration of a six month old episiotomy scar to remove a painful granuloma, probably the result of a stitch that was not removed after the original procedure

---

Possible negative experiences after termination of pregnancy

- Avoidance, denial, and feelings of numbness or worthlessness
- Anger, tearfulness, and depression
- Dissociation from body and negative thoughts and feelings
- Recurrent intrusive thoughts, flashbacks, dreams, and nightmares
- Guilt, shame, detachment, and loss of positive feelings
- Suicidal thoughts and feelings of loss of control
- Psychological problems (such as eating disorders)
- Disinterest in and avoidance of sex and possible vaginismus
- Symptoms can be immediate, delayed, or chronic

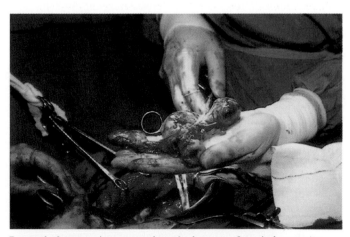

Removal of a woman's uterus and ovaries because of cervical or uterine cancer can lead to psychosexual problems in addition to the fear of diagnosis and treatment

they cannot cope with the physical differences caused by the operation, and this makes restarting a sexual life a big ordeal.

A recent study showed that 75% of women who had undergone radical vulvectomy or radical hysterectomy had sexual difficulties for more than six months postoperatively, and 15% never resumed sexual intercourse. Women younger than 50 years and those who were not sexually experienced or in a relationship at the time of the operation were worst affected. The most common problem was lack of sexual arousal.

A frank preoperative discussion is essential, and the woman's partner should be involved from the beginning. If at all possible, radiotherapy should be avoided to minimise the physical mutilation and to preserve the ovaries. At every follow up visit, all women should be asked how their sexual life is progressing, and sexual counselling should be offered early to minimise long term damage.

Discussion and management

Before an operation takes place, the full implications of the operation on their sexual life must be discussed with the woman, and preferably with her partner. To allow the full expression of fears, myths, gains, and losses, discussions should be conducted in private in a frank and empathic way. This helps to minimise the risk of sexual dysfunction after the operation.

Postoperatively, the importance of permission being given for sexual activity and of starting sexual activity early should be emphasised. If a woman has had radiotherapy, oestrogen cream should be used in the vagina. Different positions for intercourse may have to be tried to lessen dyspareunia. Clinical depression should be treated first. When the relationship has intrinsic difficulties, the couple should be counselled by an appropriately trained person.

Before surgery, some couples may have chosen not to be sexually active; this must be taken into account when discussing sexual activity before and after the operation. Good communication skills, especially good listening skills, are essential so that a doctor can show empathy, respect, and non-judgmental attitudes when discussing sexual issues with patients.

Mastectomy, breast enlargement, and breast reduction

The reason for undergoing a mastectomy is all important when the effect it can have upon a woman and her sex life is considered. Cancer and fear of it returning, chemotherapy, and radiotherapy, with their side effects, can all cause a negative body image, in addition to depression and a feeling of lowered sexual worth. Arm movement may be restricted, and the lopsided feel to the body, even when a prosthesis is worn, can be a constant reminder of the surgery and its cause. The resulting postoperative disfigurement can be far greater than the patient expected, and a thorough explanation before and after surgery by the surgical team, which should include a skilled counsellor, is needed to restore confidence and regain a good enough body image to enter into a relaxed and trusting sexual relationship. Her partner's response and support is all important as a predictor to a healthy sexual outcome. Whether the breasts were of particular importance during lovemaking before surgery can also change the outcome, as scarring and acceptability of shape can be problematic for the woman and her partner.

On the other hand, mastectomy also can be a great relief and a physical and sexual necessity for biological women who are undergoing gender reassignment. It can produce good

Minimisation of psychosexual problems after gynaecological operations for cancer

- Try to involve the partner
- Avoid radiotherapy if possible
- Minimise physical mutilation
- Preserve ovarian function
- Reconstruct vagina if possible
- Check sexual activity during follow ups
- Refer for sexual counselling

Discussion of the implications of gynaecological operations

- Explain possible risks to sexuality
- Allow expression of fears, myths, gains, and losses
- Facilitate communication between partners
- Help increase intimacy
- Genital sex is not the only form of sex
- Explore other forms of sex and intimacy
- Offer appropriate support

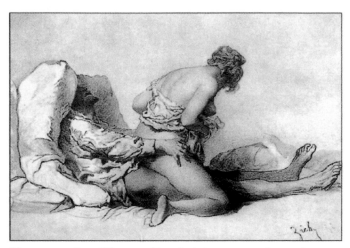

After an operation, different positions for intercourse may have to be tried to lessen dyspareunia. (Man and woman making love, from *Love* (1911) by Mihaly von Zichy)

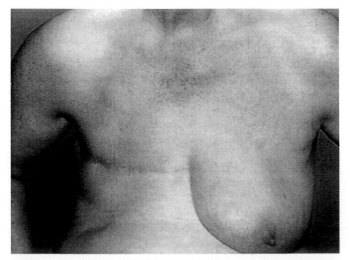

Cancer can cause a negative body image in addition to a feeling of lowered sexual worth

sexual results because of the resultant high self esteem and body image (see also Chapter 18).

Breast enlargements or reductions can offer relief and freedom from previous anxiety, especially if the feelings about the original size were reinforced by the woman's partner, but anxieties can exist about the outcome in terms of unexpected difference and scarring. If the woman is dysmorphophobic and has a fear of being deformed, however, the results may make little difference to her previous anxieties and depressed state. Loss of the expected postoperative euphoria can further depress the woman, which can greatly affect sexual expression.

The manuscript by Salerne and the engraving by Zichy were reproduced with permission of the Bridgeman Art Library. The photographs of a stoma, of eye surgery (by Philip Hayson), of female genital mutilation (by James Stevenson), of granuloma in an episiotomy scar (by P Marazzi), and of hysterectomy (by Antonia Reeve) were reproduced with permission of Science Photo Library. The photograph of a girl undergoing ritual circumcision was reproduced with permission of Carol Beckwith and Angela Fisher

Further reading

- Crowther ME, Corney RH, Shepherd JH. Psychosexual implications of gynaecological cancer. *BMJ* 1994;308:869-70

Help with sexual problems

- British Association for Sexual and Relationship Therapy, PO Box 13686, London SW20 9HZ (tel: 020 8543 2707; www.basrt.org.uk)
- Relate-Marriage Guidance, Herbert Gray College, Little Church Street, Rugby CV21 3AP (tel: 0845 456 1310; www.relate.org.uk). Also gives further specialised training in sexual therapy (a list of local centres can be obtained from its office)
- British Association for Counselling and Psychotherapy, 1 Regent Place, Rugby CV21 2PJ (tel: 01788 350899; www.counselling.co.uk)
- Institute of Psychosexual Medicine, 11 Chandos Street, London W1M 9DE (also trains doctors in the practical skills of psychosexual medicine)

9 Male sexual function

Roger S Kirby

Normal sexual function is something most men take for granted. When sexual dysfunction develops, however, stress and anxiety result, which often compounds the problem. Relationship difficulties may follow when the partner misinterprets fading erectile prowess as a sign of diminished affection. The quality of life of all those concerned often is affected adversely.[1] In order to understand why sexual function in men is so vulnerable, it is necessary to consider the relevant anatomy and physiology of the normal man.

Anatomy of sexual function

The key structures that mediate sexual function in men are the paired corpora cavernosa of the penis (the erectile bodies), which consist of two cylinders with robust fibrous walls (the tunica albuginea). Attached firmly to the ischial tuberosities of the pelvis on each side, the corpora fuse distally in the midline for three quarters of their length.

In the ventral groove formed by both corpora lies the corpus spongiosum, which also has erectile capacity. The erectile tissue of the corpora cavernosa and corpus spongiosum consists of multiple lacunar spaces, which are interconnected and lined by vascular endothelia. The trabeculae form the walls of these spaces and are composed of a mixture of smooth muscle and a fibroelastic framework of collagen.[2]

Vascular anatomy

Erection is a haemodynamic event. The blood supply to the corpora stems mainly from the internal pudendal arteries, as the paired branches of the internal iliac arteries.

The cavernous artery pierces the tunica, enters each corpus cavernosum at the hilum of the penis, and runs distally near the centre of each erectile body. It gives off numerous terminal branches—the helicine arteries, which are corkscrew shaped and open directly into the lacunar spaces. The walls of these resistance vessels consist of smooth muscle, and they act as sphincter mechanisms. When the penis is flaccid, this muscle is contracted and allows only small amounts of blood into the lacunar spaces. After erotic stimuli, however, the helicine arteries dilate, which increases blood flow and pressure to the lacunar spaces.

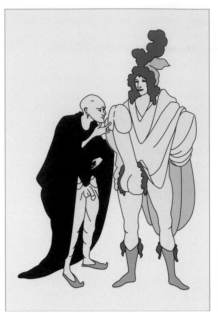

It is necessary to consider the relevant anatomy of the normal man (*Examination of the Herald* (1896) by Aubrey Beardsley)

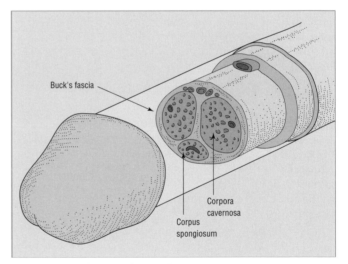

Cross section of the penis showing the corpora cavernosa, corpus spongiosum and Buck's fascia

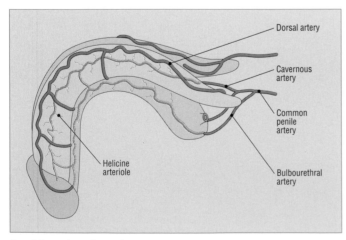

Arterial supply to the penis

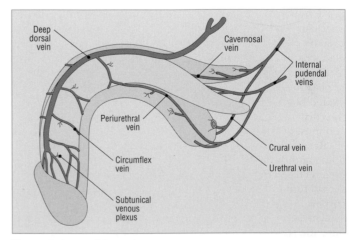

Venous drainage of the penis

Three systems drain venous blood from the penis during detumescence: the superficial, intermediate, and deep. The superficial system drains blood from the multiple superficial veins of the skin and subcutaneous tissue above Buck's fascia. The intermediate system lies beneath Buck's fascia and consists of the deep dorsal vein and its circumflex branches. The deep drainage system comprises the cavernosal and crural veins. All systems eventually empty into the iliac venous system.

Drainage of the corpora cavernosa is by way of venules located at the periphery of the erectile tissue, which form a network under the tunica albuginea. These venules coalesce to form the emissary veins, which pierce the tunica and drain mainly by way of the circumflex veins into the deep dorsal vein.

Compression of the subtunical venules by expansion of the trabecular structures against the sturdy tunica albuginea causes a dramatic increase in resistance to blood outflow from the corpora. This is known as the veno-occlusive mechanism, and it is triggered by relaxation of trabecular smooth muscle. This mechanism allows the maintenance of high intracavernosal pressure with only minor further inflow. The system is so efficient that outflow resistance increases 100-fold compared with that during flaccidity. Once erection has been established, only 1-5 ml of blood are required to maintain intracavernosal pressures within the physiological range of 60-100 mmHg.

Neuroanatomy

Three sets of nerves are involved in normal male sexual function: the thoraco-lumbar sympathetic (T_{11}-L_2), lumbo-sacral parasympathetic (S_2-S_4), and lumbosacral somatic (S_2-S_4) nerves. Somatic sensory fibres that travel via the pudendal nerves convey penile sensation. Cell bodies in the sacral spinal cord situated in Onuf's nucleus relay with parasympathetic connections from the intermediolateral grey matter of the spinal cord. Ascending fibres transmit sensation centrally to diverse areas in the brain that modulate erection.

The "sacral erection centre" consists of preganglionic parasympathetic cell bodies, whose fibres extend to the pelvic plexus, where they synapse. Postganglionic parasympathetic fibres pass forward in the cavernous nerves posterolateral to the prostate to innervate the corpora. The cavernous nerves also carry sympathetic postganglionic fibres that supply not only the corpora cavernosa but also the bladder neck, prostate, and seminal vesicles.

Physiology of erection

The penis acts as a capacitor during erection and accumulates blood under pressure within the corpora. The helicine arteries are contracted when the penis is flaccid; this creates a pressure gradient between the cavernosal artery and the lacunar spaces.

Dilatation of the cavernosal and helicine arteries is the primary event that leads to penile erection.[3] In a normal potent man, colour Doppler ultrasound scanning can detect a twofold dilatation of the cavernosal artery, as well as a dramatic increase in peak flow velocity to more than 30 cm per second. The dilated blood vessels allow transmission of systemic pressure to the corpora. Progressively, the penis expands and elongates, and intracavernosal pressure begins to rise.

Relaxation of the trabecular smooth muscle enables the filling and dilatation of the lacunar spaces, with expansion of the erectile tissue against the tunica albuginea. Compression of the subtunical venules prevents egress of blood from the corpora, which further increases intracorporeal pressure.

The penis widens and elongates to its maximal capacity, but once the compliance limit for its fibroelastic elements is reached, intracavernosal pressure rises rapidly. Once it rises

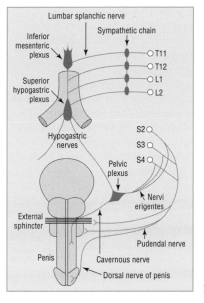

Nerve supply of the penis

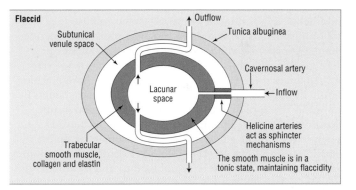

Diagrammatic representation of blood flow in the flaccid penis. For the sake of simplicity, all lacunar spaces are treated as one entity

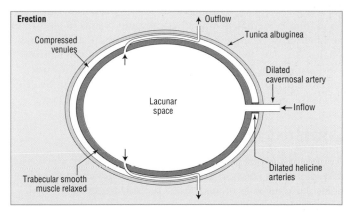

Diagrammatic representation of blood flow in the erect penis. Relaxation of trabecular smooth muscle enables filling and dilation of the lacunar space with expansion of erectile tissue against the tunica albuginea. For the sake of simplicity, all lacunar spaces are treated as one entity

above diastolic values, blood flow occurs only during systole. At maximum rigidity, intracavernosal pressure equilibrates at the cavernosal artery's systolic occlusion pressure minus the loss of pressure from venous corporal drainage.

Regulation of cavernosal smooth muscle contractility

The smooth muscle of the penis is the key factor in the haemodynamic events that govern erection. About 45% of cavernosal volume is smooth muscle; the non-muscular component is composed mainly of collagen.

The maintenance of flaccidity depends on active contraction of the helicine arteries, which, in turn, depends on phosphorylation of myosin by adenosine triphosphate (ATP). This permits the formation of attachments between actin and myosin, which permit prolonged maintenance of smooth muscle tone. This state of tone depends critically on a high concentration of cytoplasmic free calcium.

Relaxation of the smooth muscle of the helicine arteries and the walls of the intracorporeal trabeculae is accomplished by a lowering of cytoplasmic free calcium. This can be achieved by several mechanisms, but all ultimately depend on the accumulation of one or other of the high energy cyclic nucleotides: cyclic adenosine monophosphate (cAMP) or cyclic guanosine triphosphate (cGTP). Recently, nitric oxide (NO) has been shown to activate guanosine triphosphatase (GTPase), which produces cyclic guanosine monophosphate (cGMP) and subsequently triggers the lowering of intracellular free calcium. Nitric oxide is produced as a neurotransmitter substance by nitric oxide synthetase in parasympathetic nerve endings and endothelial cells within the corpora.[4] Cyclic guanosine monophosphate is broken down by type 5 phosphodiesterase. Sildenafil, a specific inhibitor of type 5 phosphodiesterase, when taken orally, thus potentiates the effect of nitric oxide and enhances the erectile response in men who have erectile dysfunction. Other muscle relaxants, such as prostaglandin E_1 and vasoactive intestinal peptide, given by injection in the treatment of erectile dysfunction also act via mechanisms dependent on cyclic adenosine monophosphate, again by reducing intracellular levels of calcium. Phentolamine, another oral facilitator of erection is a combined α_1 and α_2 adrenergic antagonist. Vasodilation is caused by the combined α blockade.

Vasoconstrictor influences such as noradrenaline released from sympathetic nerve terminals counterbalance the vasodilatory effects of these and other transmitters. These vasoconstrictor influences act to increase cytoplasmic free calcium and are important not only for maintaining flaccidity but also for inducing detumescence after ejaculation. As ejaculation is mediated sympathetically and results in closure of the bladder neck and contraction of the prostate and seminal vesicles, it is easy to see how active contraction of the helicine arteries naturally follows this event. Intracorporeal pressure therefore declines, and the veno-occlusive mechanisms reverse. This is the mechanism by which detumescence is achieved.

Conclusions

Normal male sexual function requires penile erection, which is a neurogenic and haemodynamic event. The microanatomy and molecular physiology of this process recently has been clarified. Normal erectile activity depends on intracorporeal smooth muscle function that is controlled by a balance of vasoconstrictor and vasodilatory neurotransmitter substances that modulate cytoplasmic calcium levels in the smooth muscle of the penis.[5] In view of the complexity of these mechanisms, that a wide variety of disorders can result in male erectile dysfunction is unsurprising. These, and the remedies for them, are discussed in other chapters.

The cross section of the penis is adapted from *A common male problem* by Tomlinson JM with permission of Pharmacia and Upjohn. The diagram of the nerve supply to the penis is adapted from Eardley I, Sethia K, Dean J. *Erectile dysfunction.* London: Mosby-Wolfe Medical Communications, 1999.

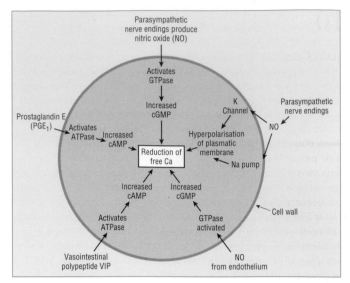

Neurotransmitter substances control intracorporeal smooth muscle contractility by modulating cytoplasmic free calcium. NO, nitric oxide. ATP, adenosine triphosphate. cAMP, cyclic adenosine monophosphate. cGTP, cyclic guanosine triphosphate. cGMP, cyclic guanosine monophosphate. GTPase, guanosine triphosphatase. PDE$_5$, type 5 phosphodiesterase. VIP, vasointestinal polypeptide

Mechanisms of lowering the intracellular free calcium

Reduction of intracellular free calcium lowers the state of tone and enables the smooth muscle cell to relax. The main muscle relaxants are nitric oxide (NO), prostaglandin E_1 (PGE$_1$), and vasointestinal polypeptide (VIP).

How erectile dysfunction is treated
Sildenafil, tadalafil, and vardenafil
- Cyclic guanosine monophosphate (cGMP) is broken down by type 5 phosphodiesterase
- Sildenafil (Viagra), tadalafil (Cialis), and vardenafil (Levitra) inhibit type 5 phosphodiesterase and potentiate the effect of nitric oxide with a consequent increase in cyclic guanosine monophosphate (cGMP)
- Tadalafil and vardenafil are relatively new agents and have different pharmacodynamic profiles from sildenafil but similar side effects[6-8]

Alprostadil
- Prostaglandin E_1 (alprostadil) potentiates the increase in cyclic adenosine monophosphate, as does vasointestinal polypeptide

1 Kirby RS. Impotence: diagnosis and management of male erectile dysfunction. *BMJ* 1994;194:694-7
2 Goldstein AMB, Padma-Nathan H. The microarchitecture of the intracavernosal smooth muscle and the cavernosal fibrous skeleton. *J Urol* 1990;144:1114-6
3 Andersson KE, Wagner G. Physiology of penile erection. *Physiol Rev* 1995;75:191-236
4 Burnett AL, Lowenstein CJ, Bredt DS, Chang TS, Snyder SH. Nitric oxide: a physiologic mediator of penile erection. *Science* 1992;257:401-3
5 Holmes SAV, Kirby RS, Carson C. *Male erectile dysfunction.* Oxford: Health Press, 1997
6 Stuckey BGA. Tadalafil: phase 3 experience. *Eur Urol Supplements* 2002;1:25-30
7 Padma-Nathan H, McMurray JG, Pullman WE, Whitaker JS, Saoud JB, Ferguson KM et al. On-demand IC351 (Cialis) enhances erectile function in patients with erectile dysfunction. *Int J Impot Res* 2001;13:2-9
8 Goldstein I, Lue TF, Padma-Nathan H, Rosen RC, Steers WD, Wicker PA et al. Oral sildenafil in the treatment of erectile dysfunction. *N Engl J Med* 1998;167:1397-409

10 Male sexual problems

Alain Gregoire

"My brain? It's my second favourite organ."
Woody Allen, Sleeper, 1973

Many men would agree with Woody Allen's implication that their penis is their favourite organ. This certainly is apparent to clinicians who deal with human sexuality and see men whose penises are not behaving as they should. Professionals, however, can become as fixated on this organ as their patients and forget that it has a multiplicity of connections within the man's mind and body—and, indeed, outside them. Our concepts of sexual problems and their assessment and treatment must reflect this fact if we are to deliver effectively the help that our patients desperately seek.

Although it is convenient to consider sexual problems as dichotomies (organic or psychogenic, primary or secondary, male or female), such distinctions often are inaccurate and unhelpful. The presence of a problem is a subjective perception influenced by many factors. No doubt exists, however, that for most men, their sexuality is a highly rated aspect of their quality of life.

From various studies in the general population and primary care, 15-20% of men seem to describe some sort of sexual problem. The proportion of men who actually seek help is unknown. For many men, this is difficult, and their presentation may be hesitant or disguised in terms of another complaint. The first and crucial step when managing a sexual problem is to engage the patient with an interested and sympathetic attitude. Problems are more likely to occur in men who are known to their general practitioner because of physical or mental illness or because of their advancing age; in such cases, an established good relationship will facilitate communication.

Comorbidity

Given the evolutionary importance of sexual activity, it is not surprising that it can be adversely affected by almost all forms of ill health. We must remember, however, that we can add to this sexual morbidity by the treatments we dispense. Iatrogenic problems are common and important, if only because they affect cooperation with treatments.

Physical morbidity

In the general population, the perceived association between physical health and sexual functioning is weak, but in the clinical setting, the relation is more obvious and several disorders have been linked with sexual problems.

Side effects of treatment

Invasive procedures, such as abdominal, pelvic, or genital surgery can lead to erectile dysfunction, usually by damage to peripheral nerves. Many drugs have been associated with male sexual dysfunctions.

Management of drug induced side effects

- Delay dosing until after sexual intercourse
- Take "drug holidays" at suitable times, such as weekends
- Reduce dose
- Substitute with alternative treatment
- Withdraw drug
- Reduce effects with adjunctive agents

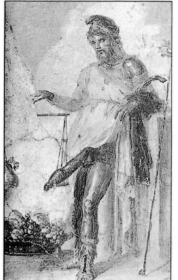

For many men, a properly functioning penis is fundamental to their self esteem. (*Priapus weighing his penis*—from a fresco in the Villa dei Vetii, Pompeii, first century)

Physical causes of male sexual problems

- Peripheral vascular disease
- Diabetes
- Multiple sclerosis
- Spinal injury
- Spinal or brain surgery
- Hormonal or endocrine abnormalities
- Pelvic disease, trauma, or surgery
- Genital abnormality, disease, or surgery
- Consumption of alcohol, tobacco, and prescribed and illicit drugs

Physical morbidity or treatments can have direct or indirect effects on sexual health

Condition	Direct	Indirect
Vasectomy	Postcoital pain from cysts around the vas	Erectile dysfunction or inhibited desire because of beliefs or fears about effects on sexuality and manhood
Peripheral vascular disease	Poor arterial supply causes erectile dysfunction	Fear of angina or heart attack reduces activity
Major surgery	Pain or neurological damage impairs activity or function	Illness, behaviour, loss of self esteem, or anxiety cause loss of activity or interest

Commonly used drugs associated with male sexual dysfunction

- Antihypertensives (such as thiazide diuretics, and β blockers)
- Antidepressants (all but a few, such as nefazodone and mirtazapine)
- Antipsychotics (all, but some are less likely such as olanzapine)
- Anticonvulsants and mood stabilisers (carbamazepine and lithium)
- H_2 antagonists (cimetidine)
- Lipid lowering drugs (clofibrate)
- Other drugs (cytotoxic drugs, opiates, digoxin, disulfiram, and antiandrogens)

Psychiatric morbidity

All forms of psychiatric disorder can lead to disturbances in sexuality, directly (through common effects on the central nervous system) or indirectly (as a result of social or psychological changes or drugs' side effects). Depression, anxiety, and schizophrenia commonly are associated with reduced desire and arousal. Mania and hypomania can be accompanied by hypersexuality. The assumption that people with severe mental illnesses do not need or want satisfying sexual relationships which is common even among professionals, however, is unfounded.

Recreational drugs

Alcohol is commonly believed to enhance sexuality. Although this is probably true for some men, its inhibitory effects on arousal and its often undesirable behavioural effects are well documented. As levels of consumption increase, they are associated with proportionate increases in erectile dysfunction, with 50-80% of alcoholics experiencing impotence. Effects are both immediate and long term, as chronic alcoholics show lowered testosterone concentrations caused by disturbance of the hypothalamic-pituitary axis.

Tobacco consumption also produces immediate and long term effects on erections that sometimes are dramatic.[1] Giving up smoking often leads to improvement. It is surprising that impotence is not cited more often as a persuasive reason for giving up smoking.

Effects of ageing

Ageing is characterised by physiological, pathological, behavioural, and psychosocial changes that can all affect sexual functioning, and it is difficult to disentangle their individual effects. There has been relatively little research into sexuality in old age, but available surveys show that some form of sexual activity usually continues until the end of life. For example, in a sample of people aged 80-102 years, 62% of men and 30% of women were still sexually active.[2] Clinicians tend to ignore this aspect of the lives of elderly people, who themselves can find sexual problems very difficult to talk about. To assume that little can be done about problems at this stage in life is wrong, however, as many causes potentially are reversible.[3]

Psychological factors

Research into factors that affect sexual arousal in men has shown interesting and clinically relevant observations. The emerging picture is consistent, although far from complete.[4]

Anxiety

Anxiety does not have a consistent effect on arousal. It reduces arousal in men with sexual problems but increases arousal in men without sexual problems. Anxiety related to thoughts of sexual failure has an adverse effect, whereas anxiety associated with novelty or threat is more likely to increase arousal. Men seem to be more susceptible to the effects that anxiety has on arousal than women.

Mood

Mood has similarly variable effects. For example, the affective response of men with erectile dysfunction to erotic stimuli is negative, but for men without erectile dysfunction, it is positive. Depressed mood causes reduced arousal, which establishes a vicious circle.

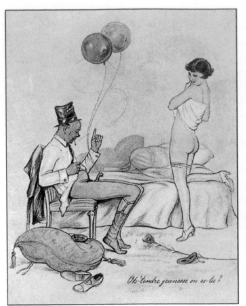

Alcohol consumption and smoking both are associated with erectile dysfunction ("Oh, tender youth, where are you?" from *The tower of love* (1920s) by Reunier)

Age related factors leading to sexual dysfunction
- Physical disease: peripheral vascular, diabetic neuropathy
- Psychiatric illness: dementia, depression
- Lack of willing partner, opportunity, or privacy
- Lifestyle factors: smoking, alcohol consumption, physical inactivity, boredom, and loneliness

These factors are common and potentially reversible

Sexual changes associated with ageing
- Decreased frequency of activity
- Decreased arousal in response to psychological stimuli
- Decreased tactile sensitivity of penis
- Increased refractory period after orgasm
- Increased rates of erectile dysfunction with age
- Decreased rates of premature ejaculation

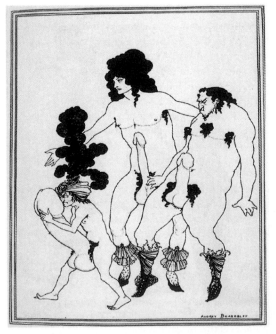

Concern about the size and shape of the penis is a common problem, particularly in young men. (*The Lacedaemonian Ambassadors* (1986) by Aubrey Beardsley)

Cognitions

Cognitions (thoughts) have a profound effect on sexual response and modulate the effects of mood and anxiety.[5] Patterns of thinking arise from a complex variety of interacting sources, such as a person's cultural, religious, social, educational, and family backgrounds, genetic factors, and past experiences. To understand these sources in any individual is interesting, but the work of cognitive psychologists shows that changing undesirable cognitions is achieved by helping the person to identify and challenge these thoughts: this is the basis for cognitive therapy, which is used to treat a wide range of mental health problems.

A common example of unhelpful thoughts, particularly in young men, is concern about the size and shape of their penis. Such concerns can lead to considerable difficulties in initiating or maintaining sexual relationships and other sexual problems. To help men challenge such concerns by providing information and in other ways usually is very helpful. Psychological approaches always should be exhausted before surgical interventions are considered, as these often have poor outcomes physically and psychologically.

Nature of sexual stimulus

Men show more attraction to visual sexual stimuli, whereas women are more attracted to auditory and written material, particularly stimuli associated with the context of a loving and positive relationship. Studies of arousal in response to these stimuli, however, show little difference between the sexes.

Relationship

Men with sexual dysfunction are less likely to perceive the quality of their general relationship as relevant to their sexual problems than their partners or women with sexual problems. Paradoxically, such men are more likely to describe improvement in their general relationship in response to successful treatment for sexual problems.

Habituation

Although politically controversial, considerable evidence shows that habituation affects responsiveness to sexual stimuli and to partners. Novelty in both increases arousal (the "Coolidge effect") and seems to be more attractive to men than to women.

Dominance and self esteem

Self esteem and social success seem to have a sexually enhancing effect, possibly more so in men than women. There is evidence that women are more attracted to more powerful or socially dominant men.

Life events

Major events such as bereavements, redundancy, accidents, traumatic experiences, or operations can precipitate changes in sexual behaviour or functioning. Problems that develop in this way can become chronic, particularly if predisposing factors were present. In some cases, health professionals can anticipate such problems and have a responsibility to discuss this with their patients—for example, giving information and reassurance about the effects of vasectomy or prostatectomy. Anxieties about the risks of sexual activity after myocardial infarction are common, and advice and reassurance must be given to patients without waiting for them to ask (see previous chapter).

The lithograph by Reunier and the painting from the *Kama Sutra* are reproduced with permission of the Bridgeman Art Library.

Thoughts and erectile dysfunction

Thoughts	Men	
	Without erectile dysfunction	With erectile dysfunction
Estimate of quality of own erection	Accurate	Underestimate
Erectile response to distraction	Decrease	Increase
Erectile response to sexual demands	Increase	Decrease

Ways of challenging unhelpful thoughts

- Am I confusing belief with fact?
- Is this belief a helpful way to think about the issue?
- What evidence shows that this belief is true?
- Am I ignoring alternative interpretations of the evidence?
- Would other people see things in this way?
- Would I apply the same belief to other people in the same circumstances?
- Am I ignoring evidence that this belief may not be true?
- Am I falling into the trap of overgeneralising or overstating the issue?

"The Coolidge effect" is so named after Mrs Coolidge, wife of President Coolidge in the 1920s, and known for her sexual appetite, who on visiting a farm was impressed by a cockerel's sexual prowess. She was told he did this "a dozen times a day." She said "please tell that to the President." When he saw the same action he asked "same hen each time?" "No, different one each time". The president replied "please tell that to Mrs Coolidge."

Friedman DM. *A mind of its own—a cultural history of the penis.* London: Robert Hale, 2002

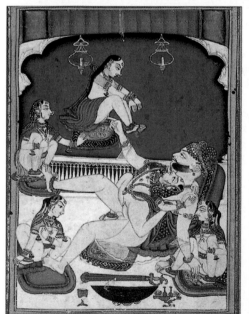

High self esteem and social success seem to enhance a man's sexual function and his attractiveness to women. (A prince enjoying five women from the *Kama Sutra* (1800) from the Rajput School, Kotah, Rajasthan)

1 Hirshkowitz M, Karacan I, Howell J, Arcasoy M, Williams RL. Nocturnal penile tumescence in cigarette smokers with dysfunction. *Urology* 1992;39:101-7
2 Bretschneider JG, McCoy NL. Sexual interest and behaviour in healthy 80-102 year olds. *Arch Sex Behav* 1988;17:109-29
3 Feldman HA, Goldstein I, Hatzichristou DG, Krane RJ, McKinlay JB. Impotence and its medical and psychosocial correlates: results of the Massachusetts male ageing study. *J Urol* 1994;151:54-61
4 Rosen RC, Leiblum SR. Treatment of sexual disorders in the 1990s: an integrated approach. *J Consult Clin Psychol* 1995;63:877-90
5 Cranston-Cuebas MA, Barlow DH. Cognitive and affective contributions to sexual functioning. *Ann Rev Sex Res* 1990;1:119-61

11 Assessing and managing male sexual problems

Alain Gregoire

Assessing problems

Men usually find sexual problems very difficult to talk about and an initial perception that their problem is being dismissed can considerably delay or prevent them seeking further help. Time spent establishing as clearly as possible the problem's nature is well spent, as it should lead to more effective treatment and may be therapeutic in itself. Likewise, talking to the partner can show a very different picture and can substantially alter management, as well as have a therapeutic impact.[1]

Sometimes quite simple interventions—information, reassurance, contraceptive advice, or an opportunity to talk to a member of the primary care team with some basic problem solving or non-directive counselling—can resolve problems that have been a source of considerable distress to patient and partner. Suggested sources of self help information, such as books on sexuality, also can be valuable.

When the problem persists despite the intervention of primary care practitioners, further help from other services can be sought, although the provision of services for sexual problems in Britain is variable and rarely enough to meet demand. Optimum assessment and treatment is provided in a multidisciplinary setting, but such clinics are scarce, so most patients will be referred to services that have a particular approach. The choice of where to refer a patient therefore will have a critical effect on treatment and, possibly, on outcome.

Classification of sexual dysfunction

The accepted diagnostic categories for sexual dysfunction described in the International Classification of Diseases, 10th revision (ICD-10) and the *Diagnostic and Statistical Manual of Mental Disorders*, fourth edition, text revision (DSM-IV-TR) do not reflect the reality of sexual dysfunctions in the clinical setting. When these classifications are used, it must be remembered that sexual dysfunctions are not all or nothing phenomena but occur on a continuum—in terms of frequency and severity. With our current knowledge, any cut off inevitably is arbitrary.

Rarely is it possible to identify cases with a purely organic or purely psychogenic aetiology. Indeed, with our growing knowledge of psychoneuropharmacology and endocrinology, the distinction between organic and psychogenic increasingly becomes blurred.

Comorbidity of sexual dysfunctions is common. For example, almost half of men with low sexual desire have another sexual dysfunction, and 20% of men with erectile dysfunction have low sexual desire.

In addition to the intrapersonal complexity of sexual problems, the patient's partner and their relationship probably have a more profound effect on sexual health than on any other aspect of health. In up to a third of patients with sexual problems, the partner also has a sexual dysfunction. The interactions between various aspects of sexual problems experienced by a couple are complex, often circular, and rarely show simple causal or consequential relationships.

Sexual desire disorder

Abnormalities of sexual desire, and indeed sexual desire itself, are difficult to define.[2] The factors considered by clinicians and patients when gauging desire include sexual fantasies, arousal, thoughts, and activity. Given the confusion over the meaning of

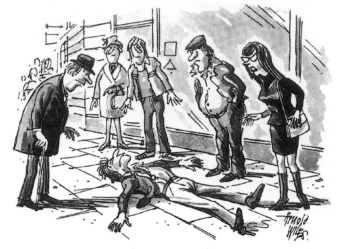

"I'd say loosen his flies but who listens to sex therapists?"

What constitutes a sexual problem?
- Physiological dysfunction
- Altered experiences
- Own perceptions and beliefs
- Partner's perceptions and expectations
- Altered circumstances
- Past experiences

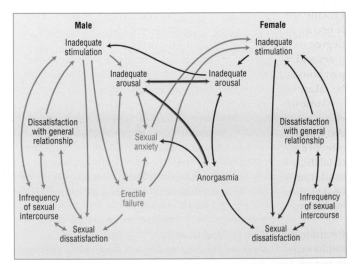

The complex interactions of effects of sexual relationships and general relationship between partners. (Adapted from Gregoire A, Prior JP. *Impotence.* Edinburgh: Churchill Livingstone, 1993)

the concept, that views differ over the term that best describes it is not surprising. The ICD-10 uses the term sexual desire, and other terms include sexual drive and sexual interest, but "libido" no longer is favoured.

Sexual fantasies, the desire for sexual activity, and distress about the level of desire in a patient and his partner all contribute to the construct of inhibited sexual desire. It is reported more commonly in women than in men (by both women and men) in the general population and in clinic populations. Differences in sexual desire often lead to considerable distress for a couple and can be a source of major conflict in the relationship.

Inhibited sexual desire often is associated with other sexual dysfunctions in the patient or partner, including endocrine factors (see Chapter 6). The lifetime prevalence of depression and anxiety disorders now is higher than previously. A strong association exists with emotional distance and conflict within a relationship, although to determine whether this is cause or consequence from the studies available is impossible. Indeed, to attempt to do so from population studies is probably meaningless given the great individual variability and the very gradual, transactional nature of change in these aspects of relationships.

Characteristic cognitive features have been identified in many cases—for example:

- the belief that desire does not gradually develop during a sexual encounter but that it must be present at the start or does not occur at all
- the belief that subtle feelings, such as warmth or tenderness, are not sexual and that sexual arousal cannot take place without intense, overtly erotic feelings.

Sexual desire in men can be inhibited by a wide range of physical factors. This can result from the general effects of illness, such as a severe bout of flu or chronic renal failure, or specific effects, such as those seen in alcoholism, liver disease, testosterone deficiency, and prolactin secreting pituitary tumours (which may occur in as many as 10% of men who present with inhibited sexual desire). Inhibited sexual desire also is often a side effect of drugs such as antihypertensives, antidepressants and antipsychotics, anticonvulsants, and cytotoxic agents.

Most studies of outcome show that response to psychological intervention for inhibited sexual desire is very poor.[3]

Erectile dysfunction

Erectile dysfunction is dealt with in more detail in Chapter 12. It occurs in 10-15% of men but varies with age, with some degree of dysfunction experienced by 40% of men aged 40 years and by 70% aged 70 years. In most cases, organic and psychological aetiological factors are present, and these must be taken into account during assessment and treatment.

Various treatments are available, but data on their relative effectiveness and long term outcome are still lacking. Although the fact that no ideal treatment exists is clear, one is usually effective and acceptable to the man and his partner. Sildenafil, tadalafil, and vardenafil—the new type 5 phosphodiesterase inhibitors—represent an important advance, but they seem to be a victim of their own success, with concerns about costs leading to limitations on prescription.[4]

Premature or rapid ejaculation

Rapid ejaculation is an inability to control ejaculation enough to permit both partners to enjoy sexual intercourse. This may result in ejaculation shortly after penetration or, in severe cases, it may occur before penetration.

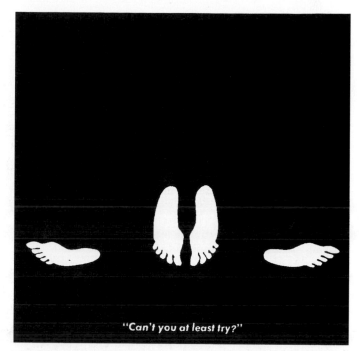

"Can't you at least try?"

Differences in sexual desire often lead to considerable distress for a couple and can be a source of major conflict in the relationship

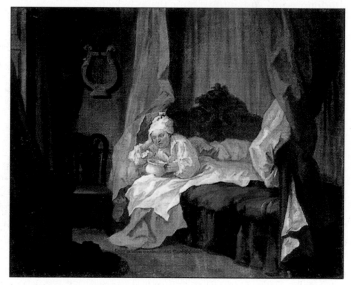

Sexual desire in men can be inhibited by physical factors such as the effects of illness. (*Francis Matthew Schutz in his bed* (circa 1775-60) by William Hogarth)

> "A hard man is good to find"
> **Mae West**

Treatments for erectile impotence

- Simple measures: education, advice, self help books
- Psychological: therapy for couples or single men individually or in groups
- Oral drugs: sildenafil
- Topical vasodilators
- Intracavernosal drugs: prostaglandin E_1
- Vacuum devices
- Prosthetic implants
- Surgery for venous leakage

Sometimes the true problem is an erectile difficulty that necessitates prolonged stimulation in order to achieve adequate erection, and therefore an apparently short period exists before ejaculation. About 20% of men complain of rapid ejaculation, and in most cases no evidence of any physical underlying cause is present. It is more common in younger men, and a process of learning to control ejaculation with increasing sexual experience is likely. Anxiety undoubtedly plays an important role in hastening ejaculation in some men.

Psychological interventions, such as the "pause and squeeze" technique, are aimed at reducing performance anxiety and improving ejaculatory control. Reported success rates are conflicting, and long term follow up suggests that benefits are not maintained.[4]

Drug treatment with specific serotonin reuptake inhibitor antidepressants such as sertraline 50 mg daily is effective in delaying ejaculation and improving sexual satisfaction in patient and partner.[5] Recent studies indicate that intermittent use can be as effective as continuous use; this should reduce the rates of undesirable side effects such as nausea and decreased desire.

Retarded and absent ejaculation

Retrograde, absent, or retarded ejaculation caused by drug side effects is seen fairly frequently in clinic populations, although many men with this problem do not complain spontaneously but simply stop taking the drug. Common causes include antidepressants and antipsychotic drugs as well as prostatectomy. Cases not associated with these obvious causes are difficult to treat.

Psychological treatment focuses on reducing anxiety and increasing arousal. Increased genital stimulation is important, and patients sometimes need encouragement and "permission" to pursue this, including the use of aids such as vibrators. One successful option for the treatment of antidepressant induced anorgasmia is the adjunctive use of cyproheptadine (2-16 mg) before sexual intercourse.[6] This is a serotonin antagonist, however, and it has been reported to cause relapse of depression in some cases.

Dyspareunia

Genital pain before, during, or after intercourse is rare in men, occurring in about 1% of clinic samples. The cause can be physical, such as genital infection, phimosis, prostatitis, or a stone, or psychological. At present, no outcome studies of psychological treatments for this distressing problem exist.

The cartoon "I'd loosen his flies ..." is reproduced with permission of Punch Publications. The painting by Hogarth is reproduced with permission of the Bridgeman Art Library. The cartoon "Can't you at least try?" is by Neville Spearman.

1 Ackerman MD, Carey MP. Psychology's role in the assessment of erectile dysfunction: historical precedents, current knowledge and methods. *J Consult Clin Psychol* 1995;63:862-76
2 Gayle Beck J. Hypoactive sexual desire disorder: an overview. *J Consult Clin Psychol* 1995;63:915-27
3 Hawton K. Treatment of sexual dysfunctions by sex therapy and other approaches. *Br J Psychiatry* 1995;167:307-14
4 Rosen RC, Leiblum SR. Treatment of sexual disorders in the 1990s: an integrated approach. *J Consult Clin Psychol* 1995;63:877-90
5 Waldinger MD, Hengeveld MW, Zwinderman AH, Olivier B. Effects of SSRI antidepressants on ejaculation: a double blind, randomized, placebo controlled study with fluoxetine, fluvoxamine, paroxetine and sertraline. *J Clin Psychopharmacol* 1998;18:274-81
6 Keller Ashton A, Hamer R, Rosen RC. Serotonin reuptake inhibitor-induced sexual dysfunction and its treatment: a large-scale retrospective study of 596 psychiatric outpatients. *Br J Psychiatry* 1986;148:217-8

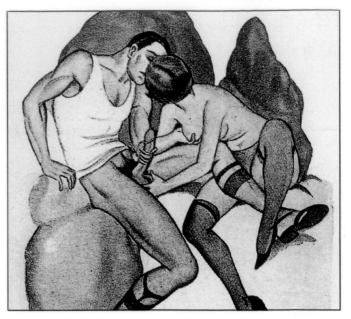

The "pause and squeeze" technique can be used to try to improve ejaculatory control. (Illustration for *The book of lust* (1920-30) by Pierre Lacombière)

Sources of further help for patients*

- *Relate*: local availability of services and waiting lists vary across the country. A fee is charged. Will usually see people individually but prefer to see couples together. Offer marital as well as sexual counselling
- *Family planning clinics*: sometimes also offer psychosexual counselling services
- *Brook advisory centres*: usually provide advice and sexual counselling. Particularly suitable for young adults
- *Urology clinics*: usually assess only organic causes and provide physical treatments, mainly for erectile dysfunction
- *Psychiatry departments*: now rarely do any work with sexual problems, as priority is given to serious mental illness, but some psychiatry departments have special clinics for sexual problems
- *Sexual dysfunction clinics*: the better clinics are multidisciplinary and can assess both psychological and organic aspects of a problem and can provide psychological and physical treatments. These clinics probably offer the best service, but few exist and waiting lists tend to be long

*List of clinics available from the honorary secretary, British Association of Sexual and Relationship Therapy, PO Box 13686, London SW20 9HZ (tel: 020 8543 2707)

Further reading

- Bancroft J. *Human sexuality and its problems.* Edinburgh: Churchill Livingstone, 1989
  Although this book is now a little old and in need of revision in some areas (such as management of erectile dysfunction), it remains one of the best comprehensive textbooks in the subject
- Carson C, Holmes S, Kirby R. *Erectile dysfunction: fast facts.* Oxford: Health Press, 2002
  A small and easily readable yet comprehensive booklet

12   Erectile dysfunction

John M Tomlinson, Christine Evans

A man can achieve earthquakes, epidemics, dreadful disease and every form of spiritual torment—but the most dreadful tragedy that can befall him is, and will remain, the tragedy of the bedroom

Leo Tolstoy

Erectile dysfunction—a more accurate description of what all men call impotence—is common. It is defined as an inability to get or maintain an erection firm enough for satisfactory sexual activity; even in young men, the rate is 7.5%.[1] The incidence increases with age until the 50s when it rises to 50-60%—not just because of the effects of age but also the effects of the morbidity of being older, such as diabetes, high blood pressure, arteriopathy that needs treatment, and prostatic problems that need surgery.

The cause was thought to be psychogenic until 30 years ago, but now it is realised that physical problems are the main causes in many patients. In most younger men, however, it is often psychogenic. Nevertheless, failure to get an erection at any age, whatever the cause, often is devastating and gives a man great anxiety about his masculinity. Many men react with shock and start sliding down a slippery slope.[2]

The next attempt at the sexual act often brings more failure, setting up a downward self perpetuating spiral of failure and despair. The impact of failure to get an erection can cause great problems between a couple and often, much misery. This may lead to separation and divorce just because of a couple's inability to talk to each other and understand each other's view. His doctor's empathy and understanding can alleviate a lot of the patient's misery, improve his mood, and increase his sense of self-worth, although attempts at suicide have occurred.

Causes

Causes of erectile dysfunction can be psychogenic, physical, or a combination of both.

Psychogenic causes

Performance anxiety

Performance anxiety does not always result in a second failure, because a single failure may happen to most men sometime in their sexual lives. It seems to depend to a certain extent on the confidence and self assurance of the man himself, as well as the closeness of the couple's relationship and the man's and his partner's feelings of self worth.

Problems with the relationship

Cooling of desire caused by sexual boredom, loss of trust, or a more exciting alternative can result in failure to obtain an erection hard enough for penetration at home but the ability to maintain one with a different partner. This can be aggravated by repeated refusals or lack of interest by the man's partner. Importantly, he will still be able to get early morning erections or masturbate regularly. Anxiety about family members, a bereavement, financial worries, or stress at work and fears of redundancy all can precipitate failure.

Psychological traumas from the past

Psychological traumas from the past, especially deeply buried memories of childhood sexual abuse, can be a major cause of erectile dysfunction.

Prevalence of erectile dysfunction in the community

Overall, one man in 10 is affected

Age range (years)	Prevalence (%)
20-39	7.5
40-49	11
50-59	18
60-69	38
70+	57

Adapted from Whitehead ED. *Postgrad Med* 1990:88;2123-4

My reaction? I was horrified ... I felt as though I'd failed, which I obviously had, [in] doing what I should do naturally, which was to get an erection. I associate getting an erection with being a man. I was frightened and I felt awful.

When I got into bed [to try the second time], my first thought was "I hope to God it gets hard." And it didn't. The second time was bloody horrible, it was horrible, it was a horrible experience. I felt awful. I felt small. I felt belittled—because something I'd taken for granted, basically as long as I remember, which is getting an erection, wasn't happening

A 46 year old architect describing his reactions

But after a little while, it got difficult between us because I think she thought I was seeing somebody else and [her] natural reaction was that I didn't find her attractive anymore. It got to the stage when it got particularly unpleasant ... she would get upset and start saying ... "it's me, I'm too fat", which made me feel even worse, because I knew it wasn't her, it was me, but being the sort of person I am, I couldn't discuss it. I just tended to shut off or we would argue and I would get out of bed and go in the other room and watch television for an hour ... I suppose I was angry with myself that she was feeling bad, but it wasn't her fault. I couldn't make her believe that it wasn't her fault that she wasn't turning me on, hence it got even worse, and it got to the stage where I avoided going to bed at the same time, hoping she would be asleep when I got there

A 38 year old teacher

Physical causes

Physical causes of erectile function are many and varied.

Management

The whole person and his relationship must be considered—not just the state of the man's penis. The patient should always be asked what he thinks is the cause, and the answer can sometimes be surprising and illuminating.

Does he want anything done? Sometimes, especially if he has no current partner, all he wants to know is that he is not alone with this problem and that it can be treated when the time is right.

More importantly to their relationship, does the man's partner want anything done? If she had the menopause a few years before and has had an impotent husband for a while, she may feel she has done her job as a woman by having her children and may not relish the idea of restarting her sex life. This should be found out tactfully before prescribing.

The doctor can help by suggesting alteration of modifiable risk factors such as obesity, smoking, stress and drinking too much alcohol. Referral to marital and relationship therapy or even basic sex education may be all that is needed. Sensate focus is often a very useful way to get a couple talking again (see Chapter 1).

Examination and investigation

Treatment

This can be done very simply in primary care.

Oral treatment
Oral treatment is the first choice now, with two groups of tablets available:

- Centrally acting dopaminergic agonist apomorphine 3 mg, which is a century old drug now available in a new sublingual formulation
- Locally acting type 5 phosphodiesterase inhibitors (sildenafil 25, 50, and 100 mg; tadalafil 10 and 20 mg; and vardenafil 5, 10, and 20 mg) (see Chapter 9 for details of the physiology).[3-6]

The responses to the latter three are good, with up to 70-75% success in producing an erection for satisfactory intercourse. They may take up to 20-45 minutes to work, but if a meal has been taken, sildenafil can take longer to produce an effect.[3] The window of opportunity for sex is 4-5 hours with sildenafil, but tadalafil's window of opportunity is 24-36 hours, which allows spontaneity to be restored with alternate day treatment or one treatment at the weekend.[5] Vardenafil takes a shorter time to produce an effect and does not depend on the presence of food.[6]

A common urban myth is that these drugs give an instant, very prolonged erection, so it is important to stress to the patient the necessity of sexual stimulation, mental and physical, for both groups of tablets to work effectively. Only minor side effects occur, as long as they are not used in combination with any of the nitrate group of drugs. (Many cardiologists say, however, that the many newer, better treatments for angina on the market mean that nitrates are outmoded).

The advantage of apomorphine is that it can be used by men who have to have nitrates for angina. It is put under the tongue and is effective within 15 minutes. Unfortunately, the success rate is not as good as with the type 5 phosphodiesterase inhibitors, although submersion by taking 3 mg three times a week for two weeks is said to improve success.

A large proportion of men does not repeat prescriptions for these drugs for manifold reasons, often connected to difficulties in their relationship with their partner or their own expectations.

Physical causes of erectile function

Vascular	Treated and untreated hypertension and coronary or peripheral arteriopathy
Hormonal	Diabetes, low testosterone (whatever the cause), hyperthyroidism and hypothyroidism, and hyperprolactinaemia
Neurological	Multiple sclerosis, spinal cord damage, stroke, and depression
Pelvic trauma (surgical and accidental)	Trauma of the prostate, bladder, rectum and radiotherapy
Drugs	Smoking, alcohol, and recreational drugs Antihypertensives cause 50% of failures because of drug treatments; these include beta blockers (try to avoid initiating treatment with atenolol) and thiazide diuretics (try indapamide)
	Antidepressants, especially tricyclics
	H_2 antagonists (some can be bought without prescription)
	Lipid lowering drugs, especially fibrates
	Anti-inflammatories (again, many can be bought without prescription)
	Non-prescribed antihistamines including hypnotics and cold treatments, especially those containing diphenhydramine

Examination
- Pulse and blood pressure
- Genitalia
- Peripheral pulses
- Rectal examination, which can take <60 seconds

Mandatory investigations
- Blood pressure
- Glucose (blood, preferably fasting. Urine dipsticks should not be relied upon)

Additionally, in men with reduced sex drive
- Testosterone—total, serum hormone binding globulin, and free androgen index
- Follicle stimulating hormone and luteinising hormone
- Prolactin—especially for reduced sex drive in a younger man

Sildenafil   **Tadalafil**   **Vardenafil**

Type 5 phosphodiesterase inhibitors

Others manage to get their erections back spontaneously; this is especially the case in men whose severe anxiety after their first failure leads to perpetuation of the failure in subsequent attempts. This group, once their confidence returns, is able to continue without further treatment.

Older forms of treatment
Older treatments that still have a place in the management include alprostadil (prostaglandin E_1), which is available as an intracavernosal injection and has a 95% success rate. Not many men are prepared to inject themselves unless all else fails, particularly if alprostadil causes a residual ache. Another form of alprostadil is as an intraurethral pellet (the medicated urethral system for erection or MUSE), which has a 50% success rate. Some men find this method repugnant, and if they are not careful, the urethra can be scratched by the applicator, with some minor bleeding. Another licensed injection with minimal side effects is a mixture of vasointestinal polypeptide and phentolamine; this is very popular with its users, as it produces none of the possible discomfort associated with alprostadil. Priapism (an erection that lasts for more than 4-5 hours) is possible in about one man in 100, and its treatment must be regarded as an emergency.

Treatment of priapism

If a man has an artificial erection that lasts more than four hours it must be treated as an emergency. The longer that priapism is left untreated, the more likely that the man will have, at best, fibrosis or, at worst, gangrene of the corpora

Management
1 Aspirate 50 ml of blood from each corpus through a 19 gauge butterfly needle into a 50 ml syringe with a Luer lock
2 If the penis becomes flaccid and then rigid again, open an ampoule of phenylephrine* 10 mg in 1 ml, take out 0.2 ml (2 mg), and dilute in 10 ml of normal saline
3 Inject 1 ml (200 mcg) of this phenylephrine solution through the same butterfly needle and aspirate a couple of minutes later. Repeat this, if necessary, every 5-10 minutes until a total of 5 ml (1 mg) of the solution has been injected. Alternatively, a 20 mcg/ml solution of adrenaline can be used, with further aspiration. The maximum dose of phenylephrine should be 1 mg, and the maximum dose of adrenaline should be 100 mcg (5 ml)
4 Metaraminol* (1 mg in 50 ml saline) can be substituted, given slowly in 5 ml doses every 15 minutes. This should not be used in patients who are taking monoamine oxidase inhibitors
5 On removing the needle, get the patient to press firmly for five minutes to prevent massive bruising
6 If none of the above works, a urologist should be called in

The blood pressure and pulse should be closely monitored, especially with patients with hypertension or atherosclerosis and those who are taking monoamine oxidase inhibitors. For such patients, facilities should be available to manage a potential hypertensive crisis, which may, rarely, be fatal

*A vasoconstrictor sympathomimetic

Constriction rings and the vacuum pump
These sometimes can be a very useful adjunct to other forms of treatment. They are very safe, but the erection should not be maintained for more than 30 minutes to avoid pain because of the constriction. Some men complain that the erection is cold because the blood used to achieve it is venous.

Hormonal treatment
Testosterone should only be given if a deficiency of the hormone is proved; paradoxically, however, many men with low concentrations of testosterone nevertheless function perfectly

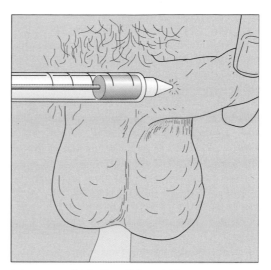
Intracavernosal injection of alprostadil

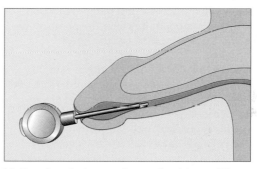
Medicated urethral system for erection (alprostadil)

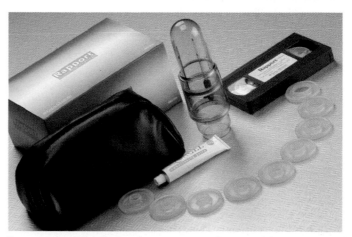
Rapport constriction rings and vacuum pump. Courtesy of Owen Mumford

well sexually with the help of an erectogenic. A great deal of controversy surrounds whether androgen deficiency in adult men should be treated, although many benefits, such as prevention of osteoporosis and cardiovascular protection, are claimed. Symptoms of hypotestosteronaemia are diminished sexual desire, sexual fantasies, and nocturnal erections; increased irritability; and often, drenching nocturnal sweats. Later, signs of loss of muscle volume and strength and increased abdominal and breast fat, and, much later, osteopenia and decreased body hair may be present. These need not all be present at any one time, and one symptom can be severe compared with the others.[7]

Deficiency of testosterone is managed by injections of testosterone enanthate (1 ml of 250 mg) or a mixture of testosterones (100-250 mg) every 2-3 weeks. Preparations such as skin patches (with up to a 50% rate of allergic reaction) and capsules are available, neither of which are totally satisfactory. Long term (six monthly) implants of testosterone can be given to those for whom regular injections are impractical. Testosterone gels also are available now and seem to be the most practical means of treatment, although few data are available on long term effects.

Surgical management

Surgery for venous leakage and microvascular techniques for revascularisation of the corpora are done rarely now, and the results are not good. The only surgical treatment of any value is insertion of a penile prosthesis. Since their advent in the mid-1970s, prostheses have developed considerably—from poorly concealed, low cost, trimmable silastic rods to prostheses with silicone that surrounds a metal core and self contained, inflatable cylinders. Inflatable devices can be two part prostheses, with a combined reservoir and pump that sits in the scrotum, or three piece models, in which the pump alone sits in the scrotum and the reservoir lies in the lower abdominal wall.

Indications for use of prostheses have changed with the development of intracorporeal injections, vacuum devices, and oral preparations. Patients who commonly need surgery are those who have had pelvic surgery or who have diabetes or atherosclerosis. Prostheses also are useful in patients who are impotent because of Peyronie's disease (which seems to be getting more common), as they correct the deformity as well as the impotence.

Cost apart, the choice of prosthesis is up to the patient. The semi-rigid cylinders stick out and are therefore not suitable for younger men with children in the house, those participating in swimming and sporting events, and naturists. The cost of an inflatable prosthesis is not countenanced by some NHS trusts, but persuasion may be possible in a particularly deserving case such as a young diabetic patient impotent through no fault of his own and whose marriage is at risk.

Operative procedure

The operation is carried out under regional or general anaesthesia. Circumcision often is necessary with many semi-rigid prostheses, so this should be done first.

The corpora are exposed and opened through an incision large enough to insert a Hegars dilator. They are dilated full length from just inside the glans to the ischium, which compresses the normal corpora. This may be difficult in patients with a fibrotic penis, after priapism, or in those with Peyronie's plaques. With multipart prostheses, all components are filled with saline and the tubing connected, the pump is placed in the most dependent part of the scrotum, and the reservoir is put under the rectus sheath.

> If hormone replacement is given, the prostatic specific antigen (PSA) must be measured initially and every six months to monitor any possible adverse effects. A rising concentration of prostate specific antigen should be investigated with ultrasonography and prostatic biopsy. The whole area of checking of prostatic specific antigen can give rise to a lot of anxiety for patients. Other factors, such as regular cycling, ejaculation within the last 72 hours, an enlarged prostate, a urinary tract infection, and many others, can be the cause of a raised concentration of prostate specific antigen—in about two thirds of cases in which an abnormal finding is noted

Preoperative counselling about a penile prosthesis

Counsel patient, with partner, that:
- The glans will not be filled
- The result will be adequate for vaginal penetration
- A small (2-5%) incidence of infection occurs
- The penis will be colder
- Ejaculation still will be possible
- The only solution to a failed operation is a replacement prosthesis
- A prosthesis is not as good as the original

Costs of prostheses

Prosthesis	Cost (£)
Semi-rigid malleable	914
Inflatable two-piece	2915
Inflatable three-piece	3437-4923

*Prices for 2005 excluding VAT

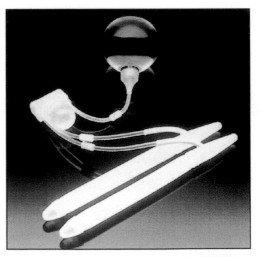

Three piece penile prosthesis in which the pump alone sits in the scrotum and the reservoir lies in the lower abdominal wall

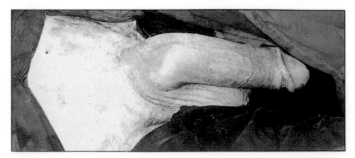

Appearance of a penis after insertion of an inflatable prosthesis, with the device deflated. Courtesy of Christine Evans

Postoperative management
Good pain relief must be provided as the operation is painful.

Antibiotics—A broad spectrum antibiotic should be taken orally for a week after the operation.

Voiding problems—If the patients have problems voiding, clean intermittent catheterisation can be used.

Postoperative use—Semi rigid prostheses may be used after four weeks. Patients can be taught how to pump up an inflatable prosthesis after four to six weeks.

Postoperative problems
Infection occurs in 1-10% of cases, depending on the difficulty of the procedure. Repeat operations are more prone to infection. It usually is necessary to remove the infected part or complete prosthesis, and, although difficult, it can be replaced six months later.

Erosion is usually the result of infection or an unsuspected breach of the urethra during surgery.

Glans ischaemia occurs with vascular compression or damage.

Supersonic transport deformity (also known as the Concorde deformity) with glans droop may be unsightly, but it may not matter if an additional glandular erection occurs.

Mechanical problems are now uncommon. If they do occur, the part should be replaced.

Prognosis
Penile prostheses give acceptable results. In many large series, more than 80% of patients and their partners were satisfied with the results. In those with Peyronie's disease, prostheses straightened the penises of 70% of men. No real age limit exists for the operation, but a prosthesis should not be inserted unless it will be used.

Peyronie's disease

Peyronie's disease is caused by plaques of fibrosis of the tunica alba that covers the corpora cavernosa; it leads to contracture and deviation of the penis and often is painful. This condition is related to Dupuytren's contracture, although the link, or the cause, is not known precisely. Peyronie's disease seems to be more common these days, possibly because patients complain more, in the hope of getting some treatment. Usually, the contracture results in deviation towards the side of the fibrosis, usually headwards, and may even prevent penetration. It occurs only in adults, and treatment is difficult. The condition is self limiting and usually does not progress after six months.

Medical treatment with long established drugs such as potassium aminobenzoate and vitamin E (Potaba) are not very helpful, although tamoxifen 20 mg daily orally for three months seems to help the pain. Injection of the plaques with steroid or verapamil 10 mg weekly for 12 weeks seems to help considerably.[8] Probably the best result is from extracorporeal shock wave therapy, which is similar to that used for the treatment of stones, with a 64% improvement in angulation and 84% relief of pain.[9] The pain usually improves in three to six months in any case.

Surgery is indicated only when the penis is unusable for intercourse. The patient should be warned that his penis will almost certainly be shorter on erection after penoplication (Nesbitt's operation). Less shortening occurs after plaque incision, but the erection is more at risk and more damage to the glans is possible. The most important feature in the treatment of these patients is reassurance and encouragement to use their erections as often as possible. The penis will not be normal again, however, and patients have to learn to live with the condition.

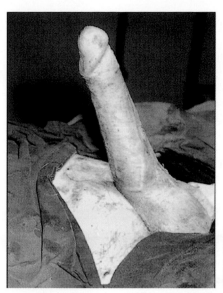

Appearance of a penis after insertion of an inflatable prosthesis, with the device inflated. Courtesy of Christine Evans

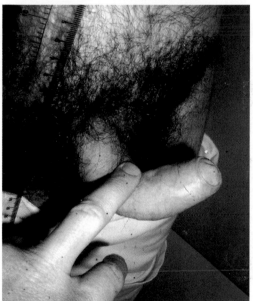

Peyronie's disease. Courtesy of Christine Evans

1 Masters WH, Johnson VE, Kolodny RC. *Human sexuality.* New York: Harper Collins, 1995: 358-68
2 Tomlinson JM, Wright D. Impact of erectile dysfunction and its subsequent treatment with sildenafil: qualitative study. *BMJ* 2004;328:1037-9
3 *Sildenafil for erectile dysfunction.* Drug and Therapeutics Bulletin 36:81-4 (Nov 1998)
4 Morales A, Gingell C, Wicker PA, Osterloh IH. Clinical safety of oral sildenafil citrate (Viagra) in the treatment of erectile dysfunction. *Int J Impot Res* 1998;10:69-74
5 Brock GB, McMahon CG, Chen KK, Costigan T, Shen W, Watkins V et al. Efficacy and safety of tadalafil for the treatment of erectile dysfunction: results of integrated analyses. *J Urol* 2002;168:1332-6
6 Hellstrom WJ, Gittelman M, Karlin G, Segerson T, Thibonnier M, Taylor T et al. Vardenafil for treatment of men with erectile dysfunction: efficacy and safety in a randomised, double-blind placebo-controlled trial. *J Andrology* 2002;23:763-71
7 Morales A, Lunenfeld B. Investigation, treatment and monitoring of late-onset hypogonadism in males: official recommendations of The International Society for the Study of the Ageing Male (ISSAM). *Ageing Male* 2002;5:74-86
8 Levine LA. Treatment of Peyronie's disease with intralesional verapamil injection. *J Urol* 1997;158:1395-9
9 Manikandan R, Islam W, Srinivasan V, Evans CM. Evaluation of extracorporeal shock wave therapy (ESWT) in Peyronie's disease. *Urology* 2002;60:1-5

13 Homosexual men, lesbians, and bisexuals

Robin Bell, Ruth Hallam-Jones

The range of sexual dysfunctions encountered in gay men and lesbians is the same as that found in men and women in general, and the skills needed to help them are often the same. That said, there are areas of concern, for patients and doctors, that merit particular consideration.

People may encounter problems when they become aware of their homosexual orientation and try to match it to their view of an ideal self. If this occurs in adolescence it may be useful to offer counselling to help with the readjustment in life that may be required. However tolerant our society may become, being openly gay still has major implications for future care and family life.

Although many gay men and lesbians are aware of their orientation from their earliest sexual thoughts, a sizeable minority do not discover their orientation until later in life, perhaps in a failing marriage and with the responsibilities of parenthood. These people require careful and compassionate counselling, especially those men who have sex with other men but do not regard themselves as gay. Some choose to remain married, and the couple may need help to reorganise the basis of their heterosexual relationship. Counsellors must be seen to be completely impartial and not encourage particular outcomes.

Homosexuals, lesbians, and bisexual people come from all the racial, ethnic, religious and other cultural groups. They may also have suffered multiple discrimination if they have a physical or learning disability, making it very difficult to access supportive health care.[1] Healthcare research in these areas is difficult because of patient anxiety about the stigma against their sexual orientation. Research suggests that these groups of patients have high health risks of suicide; stress; mental health; cancer; hate violence; and general health problems such as overuse of alcohol, tobacco, and obesity.[1]

Help must ensure respect, with appropriate, clear, accurate communication between doctor and patient. It can include (for men especially) information about safer sex because sexual exploration may present a greater risk of exposure to HIV.

Avoiding prejudice

Presumptions—When counselling gay people about sex, it is important not to have preconceived ideas about their sexual repertoire. Perhaps as many as a third of gay men choose not to practice penetrative anal sex on a regular basis,[2] and the traditional division of gay men into "active" and "passive" is not born out by experience—most gay men who do have anal sex will play either role. The assumption that the passive partner is somehow less "male" or less "aggressive" is also largely a myth. Similarly, in lesbian sex either partner can be psychologically "active" regardless of whether sex play includes any form of penetration.

Disapproval—The days when doctors tried to impose their own moral standards on patients should be long past. If individual doctors are aware that they are uncomfortable with the issues of gay sex and relationships, then they should refer the patient on to somebody else. It is difficult to focus on the relevant clinical issues if you are having to concentrate on your own discomfort and trying not to express it.

Inaccurate advice—It is unwise to advise patients on subjects that they may know more about than you do, and if anal sex is not something that you know much about it is better to admit this rather than offer inaccurate or misleading advice. Local

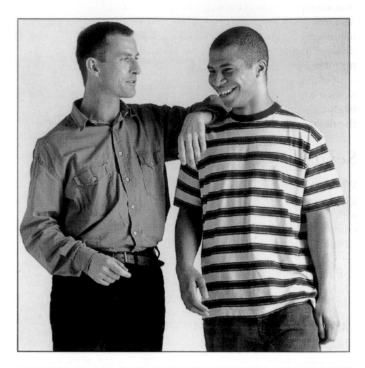

I have lived and slept in the same bed with English countesses and Prussian farm women. No woman has excited passions among women more than I have
Florence Nightingale

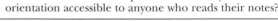

Counselling gay men and women

- Be honest with yourself; if you are uncomfortable with gay people refer the patient to someone else
- If someone is confused about their sexual orientation, try to help the patient (and partner) adjust and find someone appropriate to talk with
- Do not have preconceived ideas or assumptions
- Take the opportunity to discuss safe sex with gay men
- Sexual orientation is not always fixed. Some people—young and old—change their mind, behaviour, and relationships
- Discrimination against sexual orientation must not occur
- Confidentiality is critical. Patients need to know how much of their information will be protected. Do they want their orientation accessible to anyone who reads their notes?

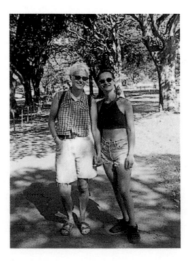

genitourinary medicine clinics should be aware of what services are available locally and which are considered as "gay friendly" and may be used as a source of reference.

Patients' reticence—Even if a doctor is comfortable with homosexual, lesbian, or bisexual patients, it does not follow that such patients are comfortable with the doctor. They may also face practical problems, such as a future application for life insurance, which mean that some patients will not wish to disclose their sexual orientation to their general practitioner, no matter how sympathetic and confidential, which produces a type of gay "invisibility", especially among lesbians. In addition, women who "come out" to doctors as lesbian seem to be less likely to be asked about sexual health issues, possibly because of the doctors' anxiety.[3]

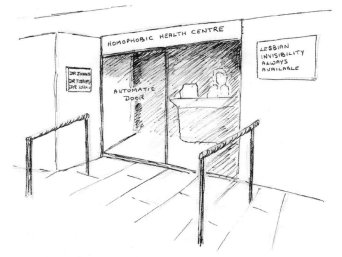

Sexual activities

What proportion of men and women have same sex experiences in their lives is unclear. Studies have been fraught with methodological errors and with researchers trying to confirm their own preconceptions. Recently (in 2000), the national survey of sexual attitudes and lifestyles estimated that 5.4% of the male population in Britain and 10.5% in greater London had had such experiences, depending on how homosexuality was defined.[4] These values are lower than many other estimates, which usually are about 10%, probably because of the method of the study.

Gay men, lesbians, and bisexuals have as wide a range of sexual lifestyles as the general community. Some live in a stable partnership and never have sex elsewhere. Others have a strong, committed relationship but with open acknowledgment that one or both partners have other sexual liaisons. Infidelity in a supposedly closed relationship is probably just as common as among heterosexuals. Single gay men, like single heterosexual men, have a reputation for having many sexual partners, and in urban communities the opportunities for this are widespread. Casual or anonymous sex can provide sexual gratification without the complications of a relationship.

Sexual dysfunctions should be assessed objectively without a moral stance being taken on the manner in which sexual expression is likely to occur.[5] Similarly, casual sex can be the reason patients, male or female, seek help—for example, if they realise that although they are sexually fulfilled, they are "missing out" on the emotional aspects that can be associated with sex as part of a relationship. Considerable distress can also exist for those who find it difficult to establish same sex relationships that could progress to becoming sexual and committed.

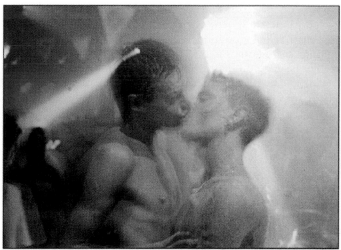

Casual or anonymous sex can provide sexual gratification without the complications of a relationship

Spectrum of activity

Gay men

Anal sex remains a taboo subject even for many professional sexual discussions; however, it is practiced widely in most communities. Sexual activity is protean in all groups, and gay men are no different in this, with much research having been done into their behaviour. Mutual masturbation, oral sex, and anal sex can be considered core activities, although many gay men do not practice anal sex. Recently, however, an increase in anal eroticism has been seen, which involves rimming (tongue-anus contact), inserting foreign bodies (butt plugs and dildos), and water sports (urination). Some couples may choose more vigorous forms of penetration, such as fisting, in which the hand and part of the forearm is introduced into the rectum.

Lesbians

Little authoritative research has been done into lesbian sexual life and activities, in contrast with the large amount in gay men,

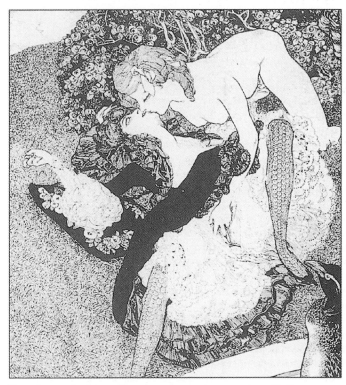

Mutual masturbation, oral sex, caressing, and penetration with fingers or sex toys can be considered as core activities of lesbian sex. ("Anything is possible!" from *La Grenouillère* (1907) by Franz von Bayros)

which was accelerated with the appearance of AIDS. This was perhaps because of the apparent invisibility of gay women. One study, however, found that the order of frequency of different types of sexual activity among lesbians was mutual masturbation, oral sex (cunnilingus), and body rubbing. The use of dildos and fisting (see vocabulary) probably is no more common than in heterosexual couples.

Watching our language

The language used by healthcare professionals when asking about sexual issues must not increase this group's invisibility, particularly questions that highlight language barriers such as "Are you married?" Questions should be made gender neutral to aid positive communication.

Questionnaires as well as posters can make heterosexual assumptions that prevent gay patients from giving the appropriate information.

Gay women and men may be under considerable stress to keep their orientation hidden from their family and work colleagues. Disclosure to others can be very difficult, so it may need to be a continuous process. Doctors and nurses must provide an environment in which the patient's history and relationships can be accepted, so the appropriate health care can be offered. If patients choose not to disclose their sexual orientation to their doctor, they may be isolated from suitable medical resources and their partners may be unable to participate in their care. People who are uncomfortable with their sexual orientation are less likely to discuss it with their healthcare providers.

Group identification

Just because an individual has a specific sexual behaviour does not mean that they identify with that sexual orientation group. Many women have a female sexual partner and yet do not see themselves as lesbian. Similarly, many men may have a sexual relationship with another man but do not necessarily see themselves as gay.

Older patients may have most to fear from disclosure. You may need to think proactively about how to give them help.

Terminology

Once gay and bisexual men and women have sought help, they often are less reticent about discussing specific sexual acts at length and in detail. It is useful therefore for doctors to be forearmed with a basic vocabulary of gay sex, although many men and women who perform these activities will lack the words to describe them, and few people of any orientation are likely to have all activities in their personal repertoire.

The terms "active" and "passive" are best avoided if a doctor needs to determine the content of a sexual act, such as when considering the risks of sexually transmitted disease. The doctor's concerns are anatomical placement and not the psychological roles implied by these words. Most gay men will not fit exclusively into either of the roles implied by the old fashioned heterosexual model, and if the words are applied to oral sex, great confusion may result. Gay male oral sex includes two sexual acts, fellation and irrumation—cock sucking and face fucking respectively—depending on whether it is the mouth sucking or the penis thrusting that is the main act. In both cases, a penis is in the mouth, but the "active" partner differs. When it is necessary to determine who did what, it is easier to talk about insertive and receptive partners to avoid confusion.

Facts and figures

- Two thirds of gay men have anal sex
- Ten percent of heterosexual couples regularly have anal sex
- The estimate that 6% of the male population are gay may be an understatement
- No-one knows how common sexual problems are in this group and their presentation varies widely from clinic to clinic
- Erectile dysfunction is seen increasingly in men infected with HIV
- A high percentage of rapid or premature ejaculation is recorded in gay men
- Retarded ejaculation is also common
- Piles and anal fissures are no more common in gay men than in the general population
- Vaginismus, anorgasmia, and low sex drive occur in lesbians just as in heterosexual women
- The apparent low frequency of sexual activity in lesbian women may be linked to women's social conditioning not to pressurise others to meet their sexual needs.

Questions without prejudice

- Do you have a sexual relationship?
- Have you been sexually active recently?
- Is there someone you would like to bring with you to the next appointment?
- Do you need birth control?
- Is there any chance you could be pregnant?
- Have you had sex in the past with a man or woman, or both?
- Would you like to ask anything?

Questions about confidentiality to ask the patient:

- Do you want to discuss your sexual orientation only with me?
- Do you mind if it is written in your medical records?
- Do you know who reads the medical records?

A gay sexual vocabulary

- B/D—Bondage and domination. The use of power play, but not pain, for sexual pleasure
- Back room—That part of a sleaze bar (see below) where sex can take place
- Cottaging—The use of public toilets as a venue for meeting sexual partners
- Cruising—To be actively looking for a sexual partner
- Fisting—The insertion of a whole hand into the rectum or vagina for sexual stimulation
- Rimming—Oro-anal contact for sexual stimulation
- Sleaze bar—A bar or pub where sex can be performed on the premises
- S/M—Sadomasochism, the use of pain in consensual sexual acts
- Vanilla—Sex that does not extend beyond affection, mutual masturbation, and oral and anal sex. This is the most common mode of gay sexual expression
- Water sports—Urination as a sexual pleasure

Problems

Female sexual problems

Like heterosexual women, lesbians can suffer from vaginismus, primary or secondary, and from anorgasmia and low sexual drive (see Chapters 6 and 7). Currently, referrals for relationship difficulties are often the presenting problem, but assessment may reveal concurrent or resultant sexual difficulties.

In her research with lesbian survivors of childhood sexual abuse Hall states that, even in this area, similarities with heterosexual women were seen. A difficulty in initiating sexual encounters arising from the experience of abuse, however, may make for more difficulties in a lesbian relationship.[6] Lesbians, possibly because of an upbringing that suggested women should not express sexual needs freely, perhaps are less likely to pressurise a recalcitrant partner.[7]

Male sexual problems

Although the literature indicates a high percentage of situational sexual problems in gay men, erectile dysfunction is being seen increasingly. Such problems are usually of an organic type in those with late stage HIV infection, although whether this is an effect of the virus or the antiviral drugs is not yet clear.

Retarded ejaculation is common in gay men and may be related to fears of contagion induced by "safer sex" campaigns.

Piles caused by dilation of an anal venous plexus are no more common in those who have receptive anal sex and usually are caused by straining to expel stools.

Anal fissures usually arise from constipation rather than receptive anal sex. If they are a sexual problem, however, they generally respond to the use of anal dilators. The medical St Mark's type is readily available, and the self retaining version is sold as a sex toy—the "butt plug." The smallest size works well if left in situ for several hours each evening. A topical anaesthetic (such as eutectic mixture of local anaesthetic (EMLA) cream) may be used on the first few occasions, until healing is under way.

Sexually transmitted infections

Sexually transmitted diseases are common in people, including homosexual men, who have many sexual partners. The ease of transmission of most sexual infections is similar for vaginal and anal sex, with the exception of HIV, which is much more easily spread by anal sex. Strong condoms greatly reduce this risk. Oral sex, although a recognised route of transmission, is considered to be relatively safe for HIV, but it is a common means of acquiring gonorrhoea, syphilis, and non-specific urethritis. Lesbians are considered a low risk group for HIV infection.

Faeco-oral spread of pathogens such as *Giardia* and hepatitis A are well recorded from oro-anal sexual contact. Minor episodes of diarrhoea may be related to faecal exposure, and are often self limiting. If they persist, stool culture usually will pick up any bacterial cause, and if the culture is negative, it is better to treat for presumed giardiasis than do extensive investigations to attempt to prove the diagnosis.

Hepatitis B, although more common in gay men, has not been shown to be spread by specific sexual practices and may simply be a marker of exposure to a greater number of sexual partners. The orthodox sexually transmitted diseases are managed as in the heterosexual community, although contact tracing for gay men with non-specific urethritis is less important given the rarity (2%) of *Chlamydia* as a causative agent in gay men. Immunisation against hepatitis A and B is recommended

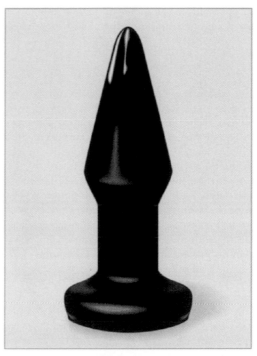

A self-retaining "butt plug," which can be used in anal dilatation exercises or simply as a sex toy

---

Infections associated with homosexual activity

- Sexually transmitted diseases are common in all people with a high number of different partners
- Their management is the same in the gay individual as in the heterosexual
- The transmission of infection through vaginal and anal intercourse is no different, apart from HIV
- Hepatitis A and *Giardia* are spread through oro-anal contact
- The greater incidence of hepatitis B is an indicator of a large number of partners, not of specific sexual practices

---

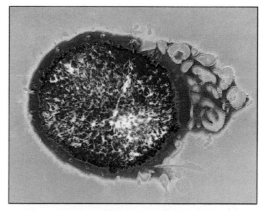

Infection with *Neisseria gonorrhoeae* can occur through oral sex as well as vaginal and anal sex

by the Department of Health for all men with male sexual contacts, regardless of whether they identify themselves as "gay."

Anal sex

About a third of heterosexual couples in Britain are thought to use anal sex as an occasional method of sexual expression, with about 10% using it as a preferred or regular method.[4] Perhaps two thirds of gay men practice anal sex as a regular part of their sexual repertoire. This means that, in absolute numbers, more heterosexuals have anal sex than gay men. Few data are published on how many heterosexual men would like their anus to be sexually stimulated in a heterosexual relationship. Anecdotally, the number is substantial. What data we do have almost all relate to penetrative sexual acts, and the superficial contact of the anal ring with fingers or the tongue is even less well documented, but it may be assumed to be a common sexual activity for men of all sexual orientations.

Anatomy of the anus

The nerve supply to the anal margin is the same as that to the genitalia, coming from S4, and the pectinate line roughly marks the division between sensitivity to touch and temperature externally and perception of little more than stretch internally. The external anal sphincter is made of striated muscle and can be brought under voluntary control, whereas the internal sphincter, which is a thickening of the intrinsic muscle layer of the gut, is made of smooth muscle and is autonomic, opening in response to stretch stimuli.

Advice for patients

- Check that the patient really wants to try anal sex and is not being pressured by a partner
- Anal relaxation is better than pushing harder
- Reinforce the use of condoms with water based lubrication as a protection against HIV
- Give instructions for anal dilatation and relaxation exercises

---

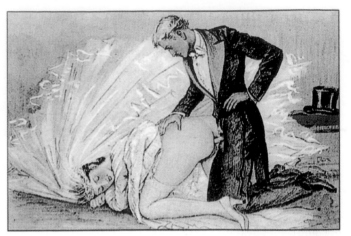

In absolute numbers, more heterosexuals are having anal sex in Britain than gay men. (Illustration (possibly by Paul-Emile Bécat) for *An up-to-date young lady* (1920s) by Helena Varley)

Anal dilatation and relaxation exercises

- Do these exercises on your own until you are confident you can accommodate a penis
- Start doing exercises in bed lying on a towel or lying on your back in a warm bath
- Raise your knees towards your chest
- Explore the perianal area with a finger covered in lubrication. Petroleum jelly is a good choice at this stage, but it must be substituted with a water based lubricant (KY, Senselle, or those provided in genitourinary medicine clinics) before intercourse with a condom is attempted. If a non-water based lubricant is used with a condom in any sexual activity it will lead to very rapid splitting of the rubber, with consequent risk of infection. Polyurethane condoms not susceptible to oil based lubricants (such as Avanti) are available but are rather expensive
- Gentle pressure with a finger moving a circle round the anus will relax the sphincter enough to be able to insert one digit
- Once the finger can be comfortably accommodated, begin to stretch the sphincter with circling motions inside the anus
- After several sessions, it will be possible to insert another finger and to continue
- Further dilation by relaxation, not stretching, can be achieved by the use of an anal dilator of the St Mark's type or a self retaining "butt plug" left in situ on a regular basis

---

1 Gruskin ER. *Treating lesbian and bisexual women: challenges and strategies for health professionals.* London: Sage, 1999
2 Coxon A. *Between the sheets.* London: Cassell, 1996
3 Morrison S. *No sex, please, we're lesbians! A feminist enquiry into the perceived gap in psychosexual services and literature.* Presented at the British Association of Counsellors Research Conference, 2002
4 Johnson AM, Mercer CH, Erens B, Copas AJ, McManus S, Wellings K et al. Sexual behaviour in Britain: partnerships, practices, and HIV risk behaviours. *Lancet* 2001;358:1835-42
5 General Medical Council. *Good medical practice.* London: GMC, 1998
6 Hall J. An exploration of the sexual and relationship experiences of lesbian survivors of childhood sexual abuse. *Sex Mar Ther* 1999;14:161-70
7 Nichols M. Lesbian sexuality: issues and developing theory. In: *Lesbian psychologies: exploration and challenges.* Chicago: University of Illinois Press, 1987:95-126

The picture of the male gay couple is by Fly Design Consultants and reproduced with permission of the Terrence Higgins Trust. The picture of gay men in a night club is by Nathan Cox and reproduced with permission of Gaze International. The picture of the lesbian couple is reproduced with permission of Gaze International. The electron micrograph of a gonorrhoea bacterium is by A B Dowsett and reproduced with permission of Science Photo Library.

14 Sexual problems of disabled patients

Clive Glass, Bakulesh Soni

Almost 4% of the population in the United Kingdom have some form of physical, sensory, or intellectual impairment—this amounts to almost 2.5 million people. Many of these disabling conditions can produce sexual problems of desire, arousal, orgasm, or sexual pain in men and women.

Sexual difficulties may arise from direct trauma to the genital area (the result of accident or disease) or damage to the nervous system (such as spinal cord injury) or can be an indirect consequence of a non-sexual illness (cancer of any organ may not affect sexual ability directly but it can cause fatigue and reduce the desire or ability to engage in sexual activity).

Two main points for consideration are how disabling conditions affect sexual function and behaviour and which sexual difficulties arise most often.

Effects of disability on sexual function

Women who undergo radical mastectomy or disfiguring trauma often report concerns about their femininity and self image, such as feelings of low self worth or fear that men will find them less attractive. In a similar way, young men with erectile dysfunction often avoid meeting potential partners because of embarrassment over their inability to perform.

"Sexuality" describes how people express their view of what is sexual. That awareness is the result of all the physical, emotional, intellectual, and social factors that have influenced their development up to that point in their life. A definition of sexuality on a basis wider than physical function alone is particularly important for people with disabilities. A person not able to use part of their body still has an equal right to full sexual expression.

Congenital or acquired disability

Congenital or birth impairments often affect all aspects of sexual development, and lack of privacy and independence in daily living means that adolescents often miss out on normal sexual experiences. By contrast, an acquired disability may have different implications, depending on when in a person's life the disability was acquired. Impairments early in life often produce low social and sexual confidence, whereas patients who become disabled in adulthood are much more aware of what actually has been lost. Although the degree of adjustment to either form of impairment may be no different, the process of adjustment is different. How people view their disability and who they see as responsible for managing the effects of the condition greatly influences their ability to cope.

Hidden impairment

Patients with an impairment that is hidden from others but that affects continence or sexual function often find the situation unbearable. People with spina bifida and perineal paraplegia often walk without apparent difficulty but experience problems with sexual function and with control of their bladder and bowel. The unpredictability of control often leads them to avoid social mixing, which increases their isolation. People with disabilities often present with low self confidence and poor body image, so doctors should not confuse the severity of a condition with the severity of its impact on the patient.

Men with cardiac problems such as angina often present with sexual problems because they are worried about bringing

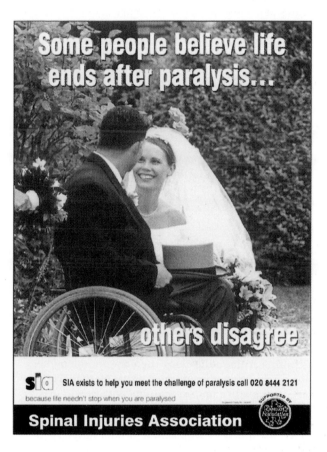

Some people believe life ends after paralysis... others disagree

SIA exists to help you meet the challenge of paralysis call 020 8444 2121

because life needn't stop when you are paralysed

Spinal Injuries Association

Key questions in cases of disability

Present condition
- Has the person congenital or acquired disability?
- Is the disability static or deteriorating?
- Is the disability observable by other people?

Effect of condition on sexuality
- Does the disability effect sexual function or sexuality?
- Does the disability impair cognitive or intellectual ability?
- Are there associated iatrogenic factors?
- Is fertility the principal concern?

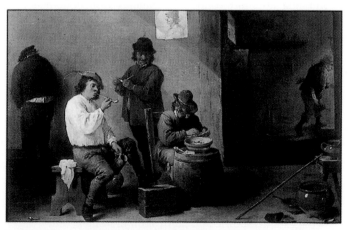

Patients with an impairment that is hidden from others but that affects continence or sexual function often find the situation unbearable. (Detail from *Boors carousing* (1644) by David Teniers the Younger)

on an attack if they attempt lovemaking. Women with joint difficulties (such as rheumatoid arthritis and osteoporosis) may find sexual positioning painful and so avoid activity.

Deteriorating conditions

In most cases of trauma, patients experience a loss that does not deteriorate, such as spinal cord injury or amputation. Some conditions, such as multiple sclerosis, do deteriorate (in either a stepwise or gradual manner), however, and this requires mental adjustment to the initial diagnosis and reappraisal as the condition worsens. Sexual dysfunction initially may occur in patients with multiple sclerosis as a direct result of demyelination of the nerve and may also be the result of indirect effects as the condition deteriorates. Problems with other organ systems may occur as well as fatigue, anxiety, depression, and, indeed, altered desire of the patient's partner. Disability services and general practitioners must address the sexual needs of not only the patients but also their partners at times of need.

Mental impairment

Some conditions, such as Huntington's chorea and traumatic brain injury, may alter a patient's ability to think in a reasoned way. Injury to the reticular activating system of the pons and midbrain slows arousal, whereas injury to the frontal lobes may result in promiscuity because of reduced inhibition. Indirect effects of brain injury, such as alteration of endocrine function (for example, post-traumatic hypopituitarism), can also affect sexual drive and arousal.

Those with learning difficulties often have problems developing an understanding of their sexual identity. This may be a direct consequence of their learning impairment or a result of overprotection by families. Parents and carers often feel uncomfortable with a child's developing sexual behaviour, possibly because of fear of exploitation or their own lack of understanding or acceptance of the child's sexual needs. The patient's general practitioner is often the person to whom family members first mention their worries or they may be the first to raise the issue.

Common sexual difficulties

People may never have had a specific sexual experience (primary impairment) or may have become unable to continue with their sex life (secondary impairment). Primary functional impairments, such as men's inability to get an erection or ejaculate or women's pain, inability to allow penetration, or anorgasmia, are more common in patients with congenital disabilities or disabilities of early onset and often are hard to resolve. Men are more likely to present than women, which may reflect cultural perceptions of the importance of sexual performance and the current range of available treatments.

Sexual function and arousal in men and women occur in response to reflexogenic genital stimulation or psychogenic desire in those with intact sexual drive mechanisms. Those with brain or spinal cord injury or whose injury or disease process affects the spinal cord experience partial or complete loss of sexual functions. They need comprehensive assessment of the level and degree of damage to the brain and nerve cord and the damage to upper and lower motor neurones (by testing the bulbocavernosal and anal wink reflexes; see Chapter 5). In neurological terms, erection in men is similar to the vasocongestive response and lubrication in women, and ejaculation in men is similar to contraction of the pelvic floor, perineum, and anal sphincter in women.

Assessment of sexual problems in disabled patients. Do I refer for sexual support?

Mainly psychological cause of problem
- Acute onset
- General relationship with partner (excluding sexual problem) is poor (refer to Relate for appropriate counselling)
- Symptoms not consistent in all situations
- Major life events (births; deaths; and potential or actual change in relationship, health or job) often present
- Coexisting problem with mental or physical health rarely present
- Men with erectile dysfunction have nocturnal or early morning erections
- Can respond to self stimulation
- Commonly aged <50 years
- Genitalia (including prostate) and secondary sexual characteristics seem normal
- Normal results from investigations*
- Refer to psychosexual services for further help

Mainly organic cause of problem
- Generally slower onset
- Good, reasonably harmonious relationship with partner
- Symptoms consistent in all situations and with all people
- Major life events rarely present
- Coexisting problem with mental or physical health common
- No nocturnal or early morning erections in men with erectile dysfunction
- No response to self stimulation
- Commonly aged >50 years
- Genitalia and secondary sexual characteristics show abnormal structure or development
- Abnormal results from investigations*
- Abnormal genitalia and coexisting health problems—refer to suitable specialist

*Full blood count; urea and electrolytes; urine analysis; liver function; and thyroxin, glucose, and sex hormone concentrations

Adapted from Sefton psychosexual advisory network

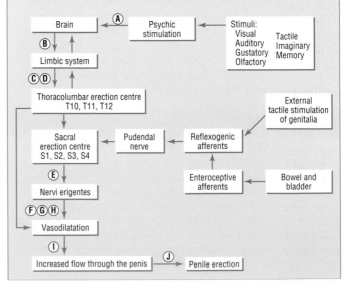

(A) Psychological factors are among the most common factors for erectile dysfunction
(B) Lesions in the anterior temporal lobe (vascular, traumatic, etc)
(C) Complete suprasacral spinal cord lesion, which permits only reflexogenic erection
(D) Incomplete suprasacral spinal cord lesion, which allows erection of either reflexogenic or psychogenic origin
(E) Complete infrasacral spinal cord lesion, which abolishes erection
(F) Autonomic neuropathy leads to impotence (such as in diabetes)
(G) Radical pelvic surgery can cause damage to the local nerve plexus (such as abdominoperineal resection of the rectum)
(H) Drugs that inhibit the action of acetylcholine
(I) Major vascular occlusion in the abdomen or pelvis, which impedes blood supply to penile tissue
(J) Fibrous plaques of Peyronie's disease and damage to the cavernosal tissue after prolonged priapism can be a major problem
In addition, many endocrine disorders are associated with impotence (for example, hypopituitarism, Addison's disease, adrenal feminisation), but the mechanism remains unclear

Causes of erectile dysfunction

Effects of drugs

Many disabled people take drugs to control conditions associated with their disability or for pre-existing conditions. Drugs prescribed for medical conditions account for about 25% of cases of erectile dysfunction, and 10% of commonly prescribed drugs produce erectile dysfunction. Overuse of other addictive drugs such as alcohol, tobacco, and cannabis can also disrupt sexual functioning.

Erectile dysfunction

Loss of erectile function is the most common sexual problem among disabled patients. Even in cases with a clear physical cause, psychological factors often are important and must be considered. With physical loss of erection, injection of drugs such as alprostadil intracavernosally directly into the penis often is the only effective treatment in men with spinal disease or after trauma, but they or their partner need to be able to use a syringe. Otherwise, erectile dysfunction most often is treated with the newer oral drugs such as the centrally acting sublingual apomorphine or the phosphodiesterase type 5 inhibitors, sildenafil, tadalafil, and vardenafil, which enhance erectile ability in up to 85% of patients. Vacuum devices, which can produce a good result in 85-95% of patients, can be used by men who do not want to inject themselves. Topical preparations are available, but these are used less often because of their relative lack of success. Patients with erectile dysfunction of primarily psychological origin may benefit from a wide range of specialist psychological therapies, which usually include their partner (see Chapter 12).

Difficulties with ejaculation

Ejaculatory dysfunction among disabled people is most common in men with spinal cord injury, multiple sclerosis, spina bifida, and transverse myelitis. Ejaculation involves closure of the bladder neck (through sympathetic stimulation) and relaxation of the external sphincter.

Patients with spinal damage often experience retrograde ejaculation into the bladder because of sympathetic damage, and various procedures have been used to induce an ejaculate. In men with an upper motor neurone lesion but with an intact sacral cord, vibratory stimulation often is used. After training, vibratory stimulation of the penis can be attempted at home. Once the frequency and amplitude of the vibration has been selected, the vibrator is applied to the penis to stimulate the pudendal nerve.

If this is unsuccessful, patients with lower motor neurone injuries can be helped by electroejaculation. This involves insertion of a stimulatory probe into the rectum to stimulate the midsacral roots directly, but it requires hospital attendance because of the complexity of the procedure and the potential side effects of pain and autonomic dysreflexia.

Fertility problems

For men with neurological impairment, obtaining semen with a reasonable sperm count and motility is a problem. The same difficulty occurs with many other injuries and as a side effect of drugs used to treat various conditions.

Women with traumatic brain injury, epilepsy, multiple sclerosis, and diabetes retain an anatomically reproductive system, but the physiological effects of their condition may alter ovulation or hormone secretion. The lower pregnancy rates reported in disabled women are probably the result of conception being avoided because of patients' concerns over their ability to raise a family and manage their impairment. Those with congenital disorders known to affect fertility and childbirth should be given the opportunity to discuss any of their anxieties with a genetic counsellor.

Drugs that can cause erectile dysfunction

Antipsychotics, anxiolytics, and hypnotics
- Phenothiazines—such as chlorpromazine
- Butyrophenones—such as haloperidol
- Benzodiazepines

Anticholinergics
- Atropine
- Diphenhydramine—such as in over the counter cold remedies and sleeping pills

Hormones
- Corticosteroids
- Oestrogens
- Anbolic steroids (high dose)

Antiandrogens

Antidepressants
- Tricyclics—such as amitriptyline, imipramine, and dothiepin
- Monoamine oxidase inhibitors—such as phenelzine
- Selective serotonin reuptake inhibitors—may cause ejaculatory problems

Antihypertensives
- Diuretics—such as thiazides and spironolactone
- Vasodilators
- Central sympatholytics—such as methyldopa, clonidine, and reserpine
- Ganglion blockers—such as guanethidine, bethanidine
- beta blockers—such as propranolol, metoprolol, and atenolol
- Angiotensin converting enzyme inhibitors—such as enalapril
- Calcium channel blockers—such as nifedipine

Dopamine antagonists
- Metoclopramide

H_2 antagonists
- Cimetidine

Psychotropic drugs
- Alcohol
- Cannabis
- Amphetamines
- Barbiturates
- Opioids

Tobacco smoking

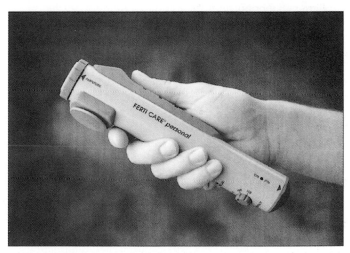

Ferticare personal vibrator—developed to help men with spinal cord injuries to ejaculate; it is effective in 80% of cases

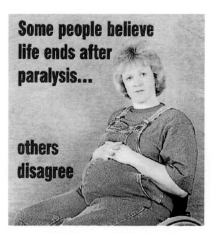

Some people believe life ends after paralysis... others disagree

Options exist to improve sexual function and fertility for people with a wide range of disabling conditions

Assisted conception

Technology exists to obtain ejaculate from most men, but the problem of semen quality, particularly sperm motility, remains. The reason for this is unclear, although scrotal hyperthermia, long term use of certain drugs, prolonged sitting in wheelchairs, and repeated urinary tract infections all have been suggested.

At the simplest level, couples can be taught to obtain semen with a vibrator at home and introduce it into the vagina with a standard syringe. If sperm motility is low (<35%), in vitro fertilisation can be useful. The process also is helpful for some men with spinal cord injury.

The recently developed techniques of microassisted fertilisation need only small numbers of motile sperm. Intracytoplasmic sperm injection, in which semen is inserted directly into the egg's cytoplasm, is more suited for men with low sperm counts. Research shows rates of fertilisation as high as 70% and childbirth rates equally as high with in vitro fertilisation. Studies are currently assessing the effectiveness of using a small specimen of semen taken directly from the epididymis for in vitro fertilisation or intracytoplasmic sperm injection.

Even in patients with conditions of severe disability, such as tetraplegia, close monitoring by a team of specialists, including the spinal injury team and urological and gynaecological services, should ensure maximum likelihood of conception and pregnancy. Options exist to improve sexual function and fertility for people with a wide range of disabling conditions. Such people do not wish for preferential treatment, but they do deserve equal opportunity of access to a fulfilling sex life.

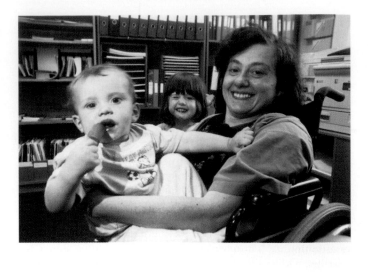

Autonomic dysreflexia and hyperreflexia

Untreated, the condition is life threatening and can result in convulsions, cerebral haemorrhage, and death

- Occurs in spinal cord lesions above vertebra T6
- Caused by increased autonomic activity after stimulus (such as distended bowel or bladder)
- Signal from the receptor travels up the spinal column until blocked at the level of the lesion
- Local vasoconstriction responses are activated, and the person experiences intense headache because of a rapid rise in blood pressure
- Parasympathetic response that tries to stabilise the blood pressure cannot travel down the spinal cord past the level of the lesion, so the blood pressure continues to rise

Management

- At first sign of symptoms (flushing, serious sweating above lesion level, nasal congestion, and extreme headache), reduce the blood pressure by placing in sitting position with the head raised
- Contact the nearest spinal injuries unit to verify the patient's drugs
- Take immediate action to find the cause and remove the stimulus
- Check the bladder for distension, catheterise immediately, or replace blocked indwelling catheter
- Check for bowel distension or impaction, give local anaesthetic (such as lidocaine gel to block adverse stimulus), lubricate, and manually evacuate after 15 minutes
- Check for and treat other causes of pressure or stimulus (for example, burns, scalds, pressure sores, ingrowing toenails)
- Sublingual nifedipine can be used to lower the blood pressure

The posters for the Spinal Injuries Association were reproduced with permission of the SIA, and the photographs were by Jim Kelly. The painting by Teniers is reproduced with permission of the Bridgeman Art Library Wallace Collection. The picture of a woman in a chair with children is reproduced by permission of The Association for Spina Bifida and Hydrocephalus (ASBAH)

Further help

Your local spinal injury centre should be able to advise on the availability of services for disabled people in the area. Spinal injury centres are at:

- Aylesbury: Stoke Mandeville Hospital, Aylesbury HP21 8AL (tel: 01296 315000)
- Belfast: Musgrave Park Hospital, Belfast BT9 7JB (tel: 028 9066 9501)
- Cardiff: Rookwood Hospital, Cardiff CF5 2YN (tel: 029 2056 6281)
- Dublin: Our Lady of Lourdes Hospital, Dun Laoghaire, Dublin, Republic of Ireland (tel: 00 353 528 5477)
- Glasgow: Southern General Hospital, Glasgow G51 4TF (tel: 0141 2012555)
- Middlesborough: North of England Spinal Injuries Centre, James Cook University Hospital, Middlesborough T34 3BW (tel: 01642 282644; www.southtees.northy.nhs.uk)
- Oswestry: Robert Jones and Agnes Hunt Orthopaedic Hospital, Oswestry ST10 7AG (tel: 01691 404000)
- Salisbury: District General Hospital, Salisbury SP2 8BJ (tel: 01722 336262)
- Sheffield: Northern General Hospital, Sheffield S5 7AU (tel: 0114 243 4343
- Southport: District General Hospital, Southport PR8 6PN (tel: 01704 547471)
- Stanmore: Royal National Orthopaedic Hospital, Stanmore HA7 4LP(tel: 020 8954 2300)
- Wakefield: Pinderfields General Hospital, Wakefield WF1 4EE (tel: 01924 201688)

Other support

- Association for Spina Bifida and Hydrocephalus (ASBAH), ASBAH House, 42 Park Road, Peterborough PE1 2UQ (tel: 01733 555988; email: postmaster@asbah.org; www.asbah.org)
- Spinal Injury Association, 76 St James Lane, London N10 3DF (tel: 020 8444 2121; www.spinal.co.uk)
- Diabetes UK, 10 Queen Anne Street, London W1M 0BD (tel: 020 7323 1531)
- Multiple Sclerosis Society, MS National Centre, 372 Edgware Rd, London NW2 6ND (tel: 020 8438 0700, free infoline 0808 800 8000; email: info@mssociety.org.uk; www.mssociety.org.uk)
- Scope (Cerebral Palsy Association), PO Box 833, Milton Keynes MK12 5NY (tel: 0808 800 3333; email:cphelpline@scope.org.uk; www.scope.org.uk)
- Sexual Dysfunction Association (formerly Impotence Association), PO Box 10296, London SW17 7ZN (tel: 020 8767 7791; www.sda.uk.net)

A more complete list can be found in the back of *The Medical Directory*

15 Sexual problems associated with infertility, pregnancy, and ageing

Jane Read

Sexuality and infertility

Infertility may interact with a couple's or individual's sexuality and sexual expression in two main ways. Sexual problems may be caused or exacerbated by the diagnosis, investigation, and management of infertility (or subfertility) or they may be a contributory factor in childlessness. Any examination of a couple's difficulty in conceiving must include overt and clear questioning about their sexual activity.

Responses to infertility

In response to being unable to conceive, many people feel emotions such as anger, panic, despair, and grief, and these may have several effects on sexual activity. The stress of infertility and its treatment may be a cause of sexual difficulties for both the prospective father and mother.

Intercourse may be avoided, with patterns of behaviour established so that one or other partner is not reminded of the fertility problem. Post-coital tests or repeated need to provide semen samples may result in a man feeling under pressure to perform, which can adversely affect his erectile or ejaculatory ability. For some men, one or two failures during intercourse begins a vicious circle of fear of failure, with anxiety leading to further failures. Partners may also develop arousal difficulties because of anxiety or distress. Some people feel that their partner seems to want them only when there is a chance of conception, and sexual activity can then become a battleground for issues of power and control.

Such stresses conspire to alienate couples from the recreational aspects of sexual expression and focus them, often obsessively, on the procreative aspect of sexual intercourse.

Sexual problems that result in infertility

Childlessness may be the result of an existing sexual dysfunction. One study of infertile couples found that 5% had a history of sexual problems.

To avoid waste of time and resources, patients must be given the opportunity to discuss their previous pattern of sexual functioning to see if it has changed because of their fertility problems. It seems inexcusable that people can undergo months or years of invasive and expensive treatment when simple questions about their sexual lives may elicit information that could spare them the ordeal. Infertility examinations should include an evaluation of couples' sexual behaviour, with special reference to frequency and timing of coitus.

Two further categories of sexual dysfunction need to be borne in mind. The first is retrograde ejaculation, in which, at orgasm, the ejaculate is expelled back into the bladder rather than externally. This can be checked fairly simply by examining a post-ejaculatory urine sample for the presence of sperm. Men with this condition experience "dry" orgasm—they feel the sensation of muscular action and orgasm but do not produce an ejaculate. This is a fairly common presentation in fertility units and can be managed medically by centrifuging the urine to collect the sperm.

The second point that should be considered is whether the sperm are being introduced into the vagina. This can mean talking in very clear terms to the couple about the nature of

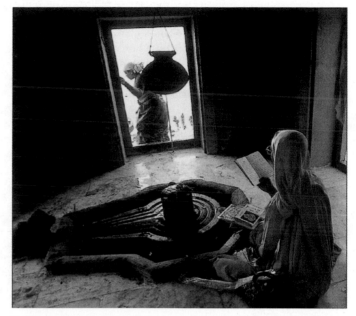

Fertility has always been vitally important in human society, and its absence can lead to anger, panic, despair, and grief, which may have several effects on sexual activity. (Photograph shows prayers being read before a lingam, the phallic symbol of Shiva, Hindu god of fertility)

Useful questions to elicit information
Taken from Read (1995)[1]

- How have your fertility problems affected your relationship, including your sexual relationship?
- Has anything changed in your sexual relationship since you have been trying to conceive?
- How would you describe your sexual activity?
- How often do you have penetrative (that is, penis in vagina) sex?

Sexual problems often associated with infertility

Male problems
- Loss of desire, with a consequent decrease in sexual activity
- Erectile problems
- Premature ejaculation—little or no control over ejaculatory response, and ejaculation may occur before vaginal entry achieved
- Retarded ejaculation—difficulty ejaculating intravaginally, or at all

Female problems
- Loss of desire
- Vaginismus
- Dyspareunia
- Anorgasmia

---

their sexual activity. Some couples engage in anal intercourse, umbilical sex, or manual stimulation alone and somewhat naively consider that their sexual behaviour is normal and should result in pregnancy.

Sexual difficulties in pregnancy

Pregnancy is a transition from one physical state to another. In the case of a first pregnancy, it is a transition from one state of being to another—from being a couple to being a family, from being a person in a relationship with another to motherhood or fatherhood. As with any transition, a sense of loss is felt, as well as the excitement of entering another phase of life's experience.

It is important to remember that pregnancy is not always met with joy and that, even if a baby is planned and wanted, some ambivalence may be present. Included in this response will be myths about pregnancy, taboos about sexual activity during pregnancy, fears about the baby and delivery, changes in the relationship with the partner, and beliefs about the roles of motherhood and fatherhood. The woman's changing body shape may cause distress and a sense of unattractiveness.

This ambivalence may manifest in sexual difficulties that are essentially psychological in origin, occurring as an emotional response to the changed or changing state, or they may be a direct physical response to the pregnancy. One, of course, does not exclude the other, and a mixed aetiology is common.[4] A combination of sexual problems may be present, and they may also occur in the period after delivery. A careful history should be taken to ascertain what is causing any difficulties.

Psychological factors

In cases in which pregnancy is the result of infertility treatment or a woman has a history of repeated miscarriages, fetal abnormality, or neonatal death, high levels of anxiety may be present, with repeated requests for reassurance or perhaps demands for scans or examinations. Apart from general anxiety, the woman may have specific concerns about body image, delivery, motherhood, changes to the couple's relationship, miscarriage, lack of self esteem, sexual guilt, and tiredness.

Myths about intercourse during pregnancy include the fear it may cause miscarriage, premature labour, or fetal damage. Savage and Reader found no significant increase in fetal problems in women who continued to be sexually active throughout pregnancy.[5] They noted that 27% of these women had uterine contractions after orgasm that sometimes were painful. Those who experienced painful contractions were less likely to have sexual intercourse often, if at all.

Obvious indications for abstaining from intercourse during pregnancy do exist, however.[6] These include:

- Vaginal bleeding
- Placenta praevia
- Premature dilatation of the cervix
- Rupture of the membranes
- History of premature delivery
- Multiple pregnancy.

Sexuality and ageing

Bancroft reported a widespread tendency to assume that elderly people are too old for sex activity and that the sexuality of men and women declines with advancing years.[7] This decline depends on three main factors: the level of sexual activity throughout a person's lifetime, their physical, and their psychological health

Sexuality throughout life

People who have been sexually active on a frequent basis throughout their life will show a lower rate of decline in activity as they age than those who have been less sexually active. Most older people who remain sexually active get high enjoyment from sex,[8] and, in a summary of studies on sex and ageing, Kaplan concluded that most physically healthy men and women

---

Physical factors associated with pregnancy that can reduce sexual activity. Data from Reamy & White (1985)[2]

- Tiredness
- Backache
- Dyspareunia
    - Pelvic vasocongestion
    - Vaginal congestion with reduced lubrication
    - Subluxation of pubic symphysis and sacroiliac joints
    - Retroverted uterus, particularly in first weeks of pregnancy
    - Weight of partner on uterus during intercourse in late pregnancy
    - Deep engagement of fetal head
    - Infection with *Candida* or *Trichomonas*
- Haemorrhoids
- Urinary tract infections
- Stress incontinence
- Vulval varicose veins

Points to consider when taking a history

- Assessment of the relationship, sexually and otherwise, and the patient's support network
- Whether the pregnancy was planned
- Previous outcomes of pregnancies (such as miscarriage or termination)
- Previous deliveries—type and presence of trauma
- Current children's health
- Contraception—past and current use and plans for the future

---

"Neither pregnancy nor its absence is inherently desirable. The occurrence of a pregnancy can be met with joy or despair, and its absence can be a cause of relief or anguish. Whether these states are wanted, the conscious or unconscious meanings attached to pregnancy and infertility, the responses of others, the perceived implications of these states and expectations for the future are all critical factors in determining an individual's response."[3]

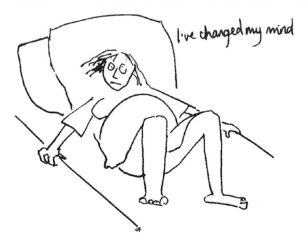

Pregnancy is not always met with joy, and even if a baby is planned and wanted, some ambivalence may be present

---

Sexual problems during or after pregnancy

Female problems
- Loss of libido associated with, for example, tiredness and negative body image
- Anorgasmia associated with lack of arousal or pain
- Vaginismus associated with pain or trauma from delivery

Male problems
- Lack of desire
- Erectile dysfunction associated with fears raised by watching the delivery, causing pain on intercourse, or fatherhood
- Premature ejaculation associated with fears raised by watching the delivery, causing pain on intercourse, or fatherhood

remain sexually active on a regular basis into their ninth decade.[9]

What form this sexual activity takes could include solo and mutual masturbation, oral sex, and penetrative intercourse. You must remember that older people may have just as wide a range of interests and preferences as younger people.

Dementia is not a normal consequence of ageing, although the prevalence of moderate to severe dementia is 1.4% in those aged 60-69 years, 4.1% in those aged 70-79 years, and 13% in those aged 80–84 years.[10] Most cases of dementia will be in women, who have a longer life expectancy and are more likely to be on their own or in residential care. Affected men tend to have a home carer, usually a spouse. These factors have implications for intimacy and sexuality.

Depression is a common feature of ageing in men and women, and sexual problems may occur with a depressive illness or be a complication of its treatment. Newer antidepressants cause sexual dysfunction, including loss of desire and anorgasmia, in both sexes. The sexual problems may aggravate the depression.

Physical health

Any condition or illness can have an impact on sexual function. For example, a woman with severe arthritis may have problems using her hands to pleasure herself or her partner or finding a sexual position that minimises the pain. Careful positioning of pillows may help with the latter problem.

Patients may find it very difficult to raise subjects such as managing incontinence when in sexual contact with another person and in solo masturbation, and the doctor will need great sensitivity to uncover such concerns. The use of appropriate creams to help with vaginal soreness—such as oestrogen cream (if the woman is not already taking hormone replacement therapy), KY Jelly or Senselle, or an aromatic oil such as sweet almond or peach kernel oil (but not to be used with latex contraceptives, which perish)—may enable a woman (and her partner) to enjoy sexual activity much more fully. For a doctor to give patients "permission" to use vibrators to help with access to genital areas and stimulation is often helpful.

Psychological health

Myths and beliefs about sexual attractiveness and what it is may affect older women and contribute to low self esteem and possibly depression. A woman who has been widowed may find it difficult to find a new partner because of the higher ratio of women to men in older age groups.

Older people may be embarrassed or ashamed of having sexual needs "at their age," and they may feel fear and guilt about indulging in sexual behaviour after having been in a long term relationship—this is, in effect, a form of performance anxiety. For women especially, there also may be family expectations of celibacy that may be difficult to counter and social expectations that older people are no longer sexual.

Further reading
- Read J. *Counselling for fertility problems.* London: Sage, 1995
- Reamy KJ, White SE. Dyspareunia in pregnancy. *J Psychosom Obstet Gynaecol* 1985;4:263

A list of further resources can be found at the end of Chapter 1

The photograph of a Shiva lingam is reproduced with permission of the Hutchinson Library. The cartoon "I've changed my mind" is reproduced with permission of Jacky Fleming from *Be a Bloody Train Driver.* The painting by Bonnat is reproduced with permission of Lauros-Giraudon and the Bridgeman Art Library

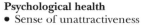

Older men and women who are sexually active and find it enjoyable. Data from Brecher (1984)[8]

People	Age group (years)		
	50-59	60-69	70-79
Sexually active			
All women (n = 1844)	93	81	65
Married (n = 1245)	95	89	81
Unmarried (n = 512)	98	63	50
All men (n = 2402)	98	91	79
Married (n = 1895)	98	93	81
Unmarried (n = 414)	95	85	75
Sex highly enjoyable (% of sexually active people)			
Women	71	65	61
Men	90	86	75

Health factors that inhibit sexual activity in elderly people

Physical factors
- Stress incontinence
- Diminishing mobility
- Decreasing muscle tone
- Uterine prolapse
- Skin tone and sensitivity
- Diseases such as diabetes and cardiovascular problems
- Chronic conditions such as arthritis

Psychological health
- Sense of unattractiveness
- Facing mortality: depression, bereavement, and grief reactions
- Loss of partner or friends
- Lack of contact with others and loneliness

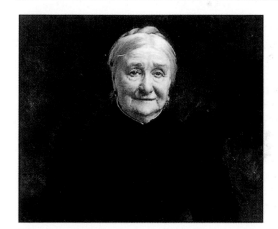

For women especially, there may be family expectations of celibacy and social expectations that older people are no longer sexual. (Detail of *Madame Bonnat, the artist's mother* (1893) by Leon Joseph Florentin Bonnat)

1 Read J. *Counselling for fertility problems.* London: Sage, 1995:104
2 Reamy KJ, White SE. Dyspareunia in pregnancy. *J Psychosom Obstet Gynaecol* 1985;4:263
3 Adler N. Foreword. In: Stanton AL, Dunken-Schetter C, eds. *Infertility. Perspectives from stress and coping research.* New York: Plenum Publishing, 1991
4 Guano-Trujillo B, Higgins P. Sexual intercourse and pregnancy. *Health Care Wom Int* 1987;5:339
5 Savage W, Reader F. Sexual activity during pregnancy. *Midwife Health Visitor Community Nurse* 1984;20:398
6 Mills JL, Harlap S, Harley EE. Should coitus late in pregnancy be discouraged? *Lancet* 1981;ii:136
7 Bancroft J. *Human sexuality and its problems.* Edinburgh: Churchill Livingstone, 1989:282-5
8 Brecher EM. *Love, sex and ageing. Consumer's Union report.* Boston, MA: Little, Brown, 1984
9 Kaplan HS. Injection treatment for older patients. In: Wagner G, Kaplan HS, eds. *The new injection treatment for impotence.* New York: Brunner, Mazel, 1993:142
10 Baikie E. The impact of dementia on marital relationships. *Sex Relationship Ther* 2002;17:289-99

16 Sexual variations

Padmal de Silva

"Sexual variations" refers to sexual desires and behaviours outside what is considered to be the normal range, although what is unusual or atypical varies between cultures and from one period to another.

Sexual variations also are referred to as paraphilias—a neutral term for behaviours formerly called deviant. They can be defined as conditions in which a person's sexual gratification depends on an unusual sexual experience that revolves around particular sex objects.[1] They are much more common in men than women.

History and culture

Sexual variations have existed and been recorded for millennia in different parts of the world. For example, early Buddhist texts contain numerous references to sexually variant behaviours among monastic communities over 2000 years ago. These behaviours included sexual activity with animals and sexual interest in corpses.

In the clinical literature, sexual variations had begun to be discussed extensively by the second half of the 19th century. The classic example is Richard von Krafft-Ebing's *Psychopathia sexualis*, first published in 1887. In this book, the author—a neuropsychiatrist—details, among others, fetishism, flagellation, sadism, necrophilia, sadistic acts with animals, masochism, exhibitionism, bondage, paedophilia, bestiality, and incest.

Major sexual variations

Exhibitionism is among the most common of the sexual variations. The usual image is of a middle aged man in a dirty raincoat "flashing." Typically, however, exhibitionists are postpubescent males up to the age of 40 years who obtain high levels of sexual pleasure and excitement from exposing their genitals to women, usually strangers, and who may masturbate at the same time.

Voyeurism consists of deriving sexual pleasure from observing others naked, during dressing or undressing, or in sexual activity. Again, the person may engage in masturbation while doing this.

Paedophilia consists of intense sexual urges and sexual activity with prepubescent children. Two-thirds of molested children are girls, usually between the ages of 8 and 11 years. To meet the diagnostic criteria, a paedophile must be at least 16 years old and at least five years older than the victim. Most paedophiles are men, but cases of women having repeated sexual contact with children have been reported. In 90% of cases, the molester is known to the child, and 15% of molesters (possibly more) are relatives. Most paedophiles are heterosexual, and they often are married with their own children, although they often have marital or sexual difficulties or problems with alcohol misuse. Eighty percent of paedophiles have a history of childhood sexual abuse.

Fetishism involves recurrent sexual urges or behaviours that concern the use of inanimate objects such as leather and rubber garments, women's underwear, stockings, and shoes and boots. Many fetishists are interested in more than one fetish. The activity involved can be looking, touching, holding, pressing against the genitals, and hoarding. Sometimes, fetishists steal women's underwear, for example, from clothes lines. In some cases, fetishists derive pleasure by getting their partner to wear

Defining normality is extremely difficult (and arbitrary), because the definition means making a value judgment and therefore labelling on the basis of how we view other people

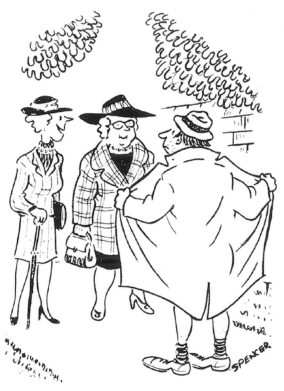

"You don't often see a real silk lining, these days..."

A case example of fetishism from Krafft-Ebing (1887)

Z began to masturbate at the age of 12. From that time he could not see a woman's handkerchief without having orgasm and ejaculation. He was irresistibly compelled to possess himself of it. At that time he was a choir boy and used the handkerchiefs to masturbate within the bell tower close to the choir. But he chose only such handkerchiefs as had black and white borders or violet stripes running through them. At age 15, he had coitus. Later on he married. As a rule, he was potent only when he wound such a handkerchief around his penis. Often he preferred coitus between the thighs of a woman where he had placed a handkerchief. Whenever he espied a handkerchief, he did not rest until he was in possession of it. He always had a number of them in his pockets and around his penis the fetishist object, such as special stockings, suspender belts, and shoes during sexual activity.

Sadism is named after the Marquis de Sade (1740-1814). This involves a person deriving sexual pleasure from inflicting pain or humiliation on others.

Masochism, which is named after Leopold von Sacher-Masoch, an Austrian novelist (1836-1895), is the gaining of sexual pleasure by being subjected to such pain or humiliation. In many cases, these go hand in hand—that is, the person can be both sadistic and masochistic (the term sadomasochism often is used to describe this). In severe sadism, serious torture and injury may be committed, and rarely, it can involve murder.

Hypoxyphilia is an increasingly commonly reported variation that involves attempts to enhance the pleasure of orgasm by a reduction of oxygen intake—for example, by placing a tight noose around the neck. Such behaviour has led to deaths. Authorities believe that deaths caused by hypoxyphiliac acts are vastly underreported or are assumed incorrectly to be suicides, when teenage sexual experimentation goes tragically wrong.

Other sexual variations include sexual desire for corpses (necrophilia) or animals (zoophilia or bestiality), arousal from contact with urine (urophilia) or contact with faeces (coprophilia), sexual enjoyment from receiving enemas (klismaphilia), or sexual excitement from rubbing the genitals against a clothed person in a confined space such as the Underground (frotteurism).

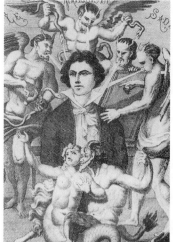

Portrait of Donatien Alphonse François, Marquis de Sade (1740-1814), ca. 1850 by H. Bitherstein

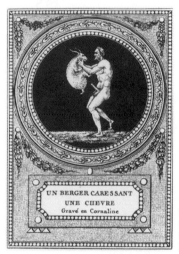

Un berger caressant une chevre—F. Hugues (also known as d'Hancarville): monuments of the secret cult of Roman ladies, Rome 1787

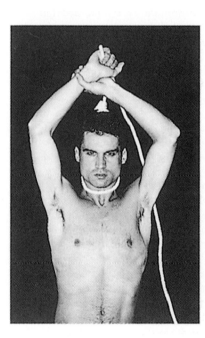

Hypoxyphilia is an increasingly common attempt to enhance orgasm by reducing oxygen intake

Transvestism and *transsexualism* are discussed in more detail in Chapter 18.

Combinations—For an individual to have more than one sexual variation is not uncommon. The most common combination is fetishism, transvestism (see Chapter 18), sadism, and masochism.

Clinical presentations

Sexual variations seen in clinical settings are only a proportion of the cases in which such problems exist. Broadly speaking, four classes of clinical referral exist.

- People sent for clinical intervention by the law enforcing authorities. These are sex offenders who are asked to have treatment to help them overcome their problem behaviour.
- People who seek help because their partners are distressed by the sexual variation and are distressed themselves because of

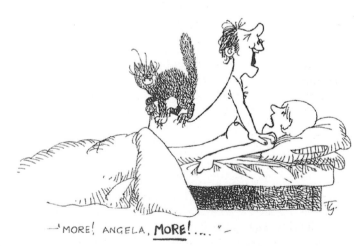

"MORE! ANGELA, MORE!..."

People may seek help for their sexual variations because their partners are distressed by the variation

their partner's distress. They have stable or long term relationships.

- People who seek help for their sexual variations because they are distressed by them. These include people who worry that they might commit illegal or embarrassing acts. Many are distressed by acts they see as "unnatural" or are afraid that they may endanger their life or their career.
- People who present with frank sexual dysfunction. They report erectile difficulties or other dysfunctions that usually are secondary to strong variant desires and reliance on these for arousal. For example, a man may find that he is unable to sustain an erection for sexual intercourse with his partner unless he has contact with, for example, a leather garment.

Assessment

Clinical assessment in these cases needs to be comprehensive, with information elicited about a number of aspects. Such a detailed assessment gives the clinician a full picture of the problem and allows them to plan a suitable intervention.

Treatment

If the goal of treatment is to eliminate the sexual variation alone, success is likely to be limited. Control may be achieved, but this needs to be supplemented with gains in other, more acceptable, sexual behaviours. In practice, this means that any treatment programme that includes an attempt to get rid of the variation must also include enhancement of other outlets. Other sexual anxieties or skills deficits need to be addressed.

Incorporation

An alternative to elimination is to incorporate the variation in a controlled way into the person's sexual repertoire. This is especially so when people's partners are distressed by the dominant role of the variation in their sexual behaviour. Obviously, this is not possible if the variation is unacceptable, such as paedophilia. The variation must also be something the partner can tolerate in a limited way.

In practice, the therapist will use a multifaceted therapy programme. One aspect of such a programme is conventional sex therapy that aims to enhance the sexual relationship. In further joint work, the couple is helped to reduce systematically the role of the variation in their sexual relationship. For example, a man with a rubber or leather fetish may be asked to wear only a leather arm band during sex. Similarly, temporal control may be introduced, with a timetable approach. The couple agrees, for example, to use the fetish object in their sexual relations on certain days of the week only.

Group therapy

Some clinics operate group therapy programmes. These are most commonly used for sex offenders. The programmes involve group processes and group learning.

Chemical treatment

For those with serious difficulties, chemical treatment is sometimes considered. Reduction of the sex drive through drugs will, of course, reduce the problematic behaviour, but its effectiveness is not selective: the drive is dampened down in total—not just the desire for the variant behaviour. Drugs often used are medroxyprogesterone acetate and cyproterone acetate.

Orgasmic reconditioning

This approach has been used since the 1970s, and its main feature is the reinforcement of conventional arousal and desires.

Areas to be explored in assessment of sexual variations

- Variant arousal
- Sexual fantasies
- Problems in arousal in relation to conventional stimuli, for example, with consenting adult partners
- Anxiety about conventional sexual activity
- Anxiety about social interaction with adults, especially those of the same age group who are potential sexual partners
- Difficulties with social interactions
- Problems with conventional social activity
- Problems with the patient's gender role

Treatment of sexual variations is difficult. After careful assessment, treatment goals must be established, and, to achieve these, a comprehensive therapeutic package is usually needed. Focusing on the variant arousal is only one aspect of treatment, and therapy that takes this as the sole focus is rarely successful

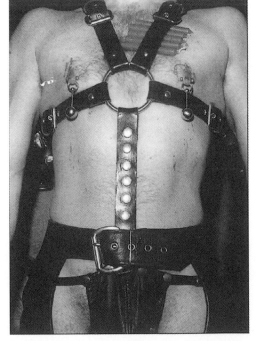

In couple therapy, a man with a leather fetish may be encouraged to reduce his use of the fetish to a level more acceptable to his partner

Typically, the patient is asked to masturbate with his variant fantasy and then when orgasm is imminent (the point of no return) to switch to a fantasy of a conventional sexual stimulus or behaviour. The ensuing orgasm then powerfully reinforces the conventional desire. In succeeding sessions (which the client carries out in privacy), the point when the switching is made is brought forward so that, eventually, the entire sequence takes place to conventional fantasies.

Aversion therapy
Electrical aversion involves the repeated pairing of the variant stimulus (such as a picture projected on a screen) with an unpleasant stimulus (an electric shock). The use of this procedure was common 20-30 years ago but now is used rarely.

A related procedure to electrical aversion is covert sensitisation. In this, the aversion is covert and imagined. The person is asked to fantasise a sequence of events involving their variant behaviour and, at a crucial point of the sequence, to imagine a powerful aversive scene. For example, a paedophiliac might be asked to imagine the appearance of a police officer at the point of his approaching a child in his sequence of images. The aversive scenes are agreed in advance and, typically, more than one aversive consequence is used.

1 Masters WH, Johnson VE, Kolodny RC. *Human sexuality*. 5th ed. New York: Harper Collins, 1995.

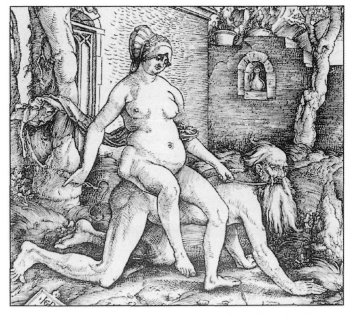

With orgasmic reconditioning, a man is asked to change his variant fantasy to one of conventional sexual behaviour while masturbating. (Detail of *Phyllis riding Aristotle* (1513) by Hans Baldung Grien)

The photograph of a man wearing leather gear, by Gordon Rainsford, is reproduced with permission of Gaze International. The cartoon "You don't often see a real silk lining..." is reproduced with permission of Punch Publications. The cartoon "More, Angela, more" is reproduced with permission of Tony Goffe.

17 Sex aids

Margot Huish, Christopher Headon

Sex aids vary from mechanical aids used to produce orgasms, such as vibrators, through visual aids for pleasure and masturbation, such as pornographic materials (books, magazines, videos and digital video discs (DVDs), films, and the internet), to specialist clothing for role play and variational sex. Aids to produce and maintain an erection are dealt with in other chapters, as are aids for production of ejaculate in men with spinal injuries. This section describes sex aids for pleasure and stimulation, and the medical problems that they can cause.

Aids for sex are many and varied, and specialist evenings and parties can be included, such as role play and fetishist parties, at which participants can dress to express gender, role, and preference (for example, rubber or bondage), which may include sexual interest. Foam evenings offer the participants the chance to party in a room filled with foam, which obscures them and anonymises any physical contact, sexual or otherwise.

Standard mechanical aids

Vibrators are used for clitoral, vaginal, penile, and anal stimulation. They can be battery operated or mains driven, in various materials (metal, silicone, polyvinylchloride (PVC)), and phallic in shape or in various other shapes for external or internal stimulation. Finger vibrators are worn over the finger like a sleeve or ring and give focused vibration with, literally, fingertip control.

Love eggs can be inserted into the vagina or rectum and the vibration within them triggered by remote control. Wires must be safely housed within the device, as they could traumatise tissue or cause an electric shock if they were pulled loose. Vibrators made to plug into car cigarette lighters could prove hazardous if used while driving. They can be used with lubrication for general pleasure and ease of entry, and they also can be used through soft materials, such as silk, to ease the intensity of external vibration. G spot vibrators are curved for focused stimulation of the anterior wall of the vagina, and men can use them as prostate massagers. Pouch vibrators have spikes or bumps, are strap on and hands free, and stimulate by vibrating against the vulva.

Dildos can be used for clitoral, vaginal, or anal stimulation. These are non-vibrating, mostly phallic shaped devices (with a flared base for anal use to prevent them being sucked inside in sex play), manufactured from latex and other materials, which are hand held or strapped on to a harness. They also are available with suction pads to be stuck onto walls or the floor for penetration. Clearly, these are visually exciting as well as physically exciting. Dangers include the tearing of vaginal and anal linings through overenthusiastic use, possibly under the influence of "poppers," which seem to reduce the perception of pain (see below). Some lubrication (mainly for anal sex) includes lidocaine gel, and the numbing effect can increase the risk of injury. In addition, a risk of infection exists if dildos are shared between partners. Accident and emergency departments have encountered patients who have used coat hangers, bananas, light bulbs, and bottles as dildos and were too embarrassed to visit their general practitioner.

Inflatable dolls—A life size male or female plastic companion can be used for sex and never refuses any request. Rubber vaginas and anuses are equally inviting and tolerant.

Ticklers are attached to a condom or erect penis to enhance clitoral and vaginal stimulation.

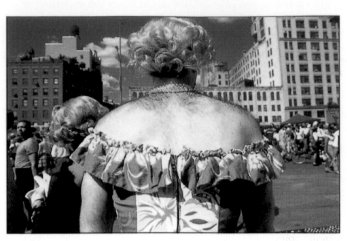
Participants can dress to express gender and role

Infantilism uses objects, clothing, and acts that relate to children. Adult sized nappies, bottles, and baby wear can be bought through the internet or from specialist shops, and users can wet and soil their nappies, which can be experienced as erotic or sexually stimulating. Services are offered by "nannies" in rooms with adult sized nursery furniture, and the relationship between adult and "baby" often enters the submissive or dominant sadomasochistic games of the angry parent or naughty baby

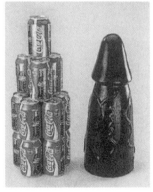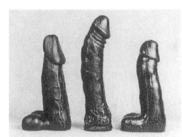
The dangers of using dildos include the tearing of vaginal or anal linings through overenthusiastic use

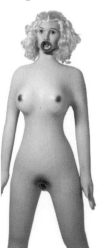
A life size plastic companion never refuses any request

64

Aids in sadomasochistic sex

Although "rough" or sadomasochistic sex is a separate category, obviously it has some crossover into more regular forms of sexual activity.

Mechanical aids

Butt plugs (see page 51) are devices that are inserted into the anus to stretch it and give a sense of anal fullness. They are generally rubber, sometimes stainless steel or leather, and are usually conical but sometimes round in shape. Occasionally, they are attached to a harness or rubber pants and sometimes are used in preparation for insertion of a larger dildo or fist.

Anal beads (pearl necklace or love balls) are connected by a cord and can be inserted into the anus then gradually withdrawn before and during orgasm.

Duck billed specula are gynaecological instruments that are effectively reverse pliers and can be used for anal enlargement. They may be painful and dangerous in inexpert hands.

Nipple clamps are attached to the nipple to produce painful or pleasurable "highs" through the release of endorphins. They usually come with a spring or screw bar and mainly are padded with rubber. Rarely, they are tubing clamps that are screwed down on the nipple. They can also have vibrating pads attached, which are wired to a battery. A clothes peg is an example of a simple nipple clamp.

Cock rings generally are made of metal, rubber, or leather and fit firmly round the base of the penis or can include the scrotum. They act as a constraint or ligature. Openable rings are preferable for safety. Rings should be removed if any sign of pain or swelling appears, and they should not be left on for more than about 30 minutes.

Ball toys are the wide range of toys available for playing with testicles, such as straps, stretchers, and weights. With enough weights, the scrotum and vas can be stretched to great lengths.

Toys used in sadomasochistic sex

Gags represent the surrender of the faculty of speech and show deep submission. They are made in a wide range of shapes. The dangers of suffocation mean recreational drugs must not used in conjunction with these devices.

Hoods and helmets in leather or rubber have important psychological effects—by removing a person's ability to see, hear, taste, or smell, they achieve the sensation of the head being separated from the body.

Blindfolds are used to block vision to allow greater vulnerability and concentration and encourage a sense of the unexpected.

Hospital restraints such as strait jackets, bed or table restraints and splints and bandages may be used.

In *sleep sacks and body bags,* the body is held within a dark and restrictive place. The body can be "mummified" with the use of cling film and "gaffa" tape (strong woven adhesive tape).

Bondage gear includes handcuffs, ankle restraints, ropes, and chains. Genital bondage for men includes cock rings (see above), cages, sheaths, and chastity belts (also for women).

Piercing of genitals, nipples, and other body parts

Thin needles can be inserted into the penis or labia to provide physical and visual stimulation, but more usual is the insertion of body jewellery such as rings, which can be pulled or have a weight attached to them. Piercings have become fashionable outside the sadomasochistic community, especially rings or

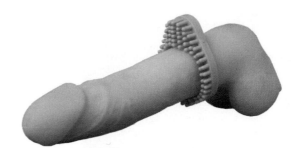

Ticklers are attached to the penis to enhance clitoral and vaginal stimulation

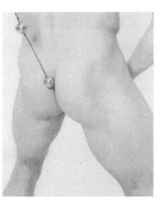

"Love balls" can be inserted into the anus

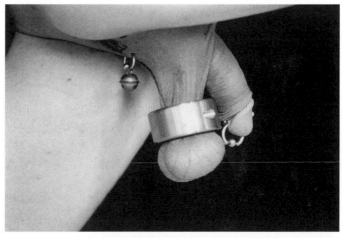

With sufficient weight, the scrotum and vas can be stretched to great lengths

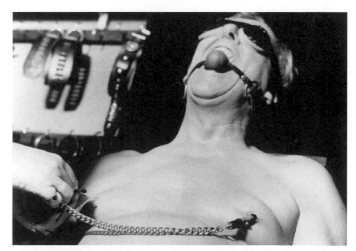

Other sexual aids include gaining sexual pleasure from suffering pain and humiliation (masochism)

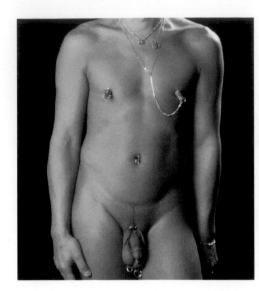

Nipple, naval, pubic, Prince Albert, and two scrotal piercings. Each nipple has two horizontal and vertical piercings

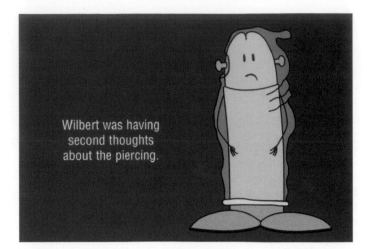

Wilbert was having second thoughts about the piercing.

Problems occur with a punctured condom

studs through the nose, lips, ears, eyebrows, tongue, umbilicus, and genitalia.

Regular cleaning of piercings with chlorhexidine gluconate 4% solution (Savlon) helps prevent infection, but if a piercing does get infected, usually with *Staphylococcus aureus* or *Escherichia coli*, the patient should not be advised to remove it, as the hole will close over and fibrose. Tea tree oil can be used first, but if this is not effective, a five day course of an antibiotic such as flucloxacillin, or a broad spectrum antibiotic as appropriate, should be given and the cleaning continued at least twice a day. Unfortunately, patients often are too embarrassed to show a problematic ring or bar bell in an unusual place on the body to their general practitioner. Problems can arise with a punctured condom.

Some writers link the psychology of piercing with the desire to find roots in the primitive and have a sense of belonging to a special tribe. The history of body piercing or adornment in African and Polynesian tribes is long and well respected.

Bondage
Restraints are used to exercise regulation and control. Many devices and practices fall into this category, and problems can arise with any of them. Fettering suggests the historical background of the jail, with the prisoner being submissive and in abject humility. Although restraints used in bondage and discipline sessions are sometimes used interchangeably in sadomasochistic sex, a useful distinction in motivation can be made. Generally, bondage is involved in practices with domination, role playing, and humiliation but includes little or no pain, unlike flagellation.

Flagellation and beating
Devotees of flagellation inflict beatings for sexually stimulating torture and punishment. Practices include beating the feet (a form of punishment called "bastinado"), spanking, caning, birching, and belting. An accompanying range of sexual furniture is available, such as wooden horses, crosses, stocks, and suspending equipment. Specific clothing made of tight rubber also may be used to heighten erotic sensation.

Other sadomasochistic games
Enemas and forced feeding through orogastric or nasogastric tubes may be used for control and heightened awareness. Enthusiastic overuse has obvious dangers.

Breath control games (asphyxiaphilia) involve restriction of the oxygen supply to the brain to enhance orgasms. This can be achieved simply with a plastic bag over the head or in more complex ways, for example, with a gas mask with a blocked air supply.

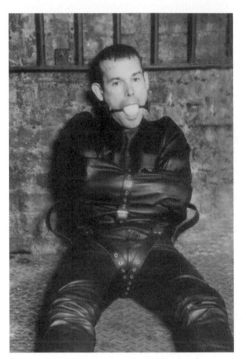

Man in strait jacket with ball gag

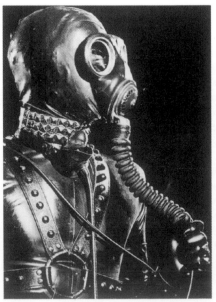

Breath control games involve restriction of the oxygen supply to the brain. Death is not uncommon

Abrasion—Some men find benefit in stimulating the surface of the body with abrasive materials, and this may become a necessary part of sexual stimulation for orgasm to occur.

Death is not uncommon. Autoerotic asphyxiation is called "solo play" and can be the most dangerous sex game employed. Sensual pleasure may be gained from the constriction itself, as well as from the excitement of danger. Some well publicised deaths from this have occurred in the past few years. After vasovagal attacks, fits are the next most common medical emergency, and it has been suggested that they can cause cumulative brain damage if regularly induced.

Medical aspects of sadomasochistic sex

It is crucial for a medical practitioner to be sensitive to the meanings that the various aspects of sadomasochistic play have for a patient. Bruises found on routine examination might cause a doctor anxiety but not worry the patient, who has willingly received them. The practices of "yellow" sex (playing with urine (urolagnia),"brown" sex (playing with faeces), and "roman shower" (emetophilia (playing with vomit)) might arouse concern about the risk of infection, but the patient is expressing deep psychic and relational needs.

In ethical terms, sadomasochistic play should be consensual, safe, and sane—you can hurt but not harm. The last point ties in with "the spanner case."

Pornography, the internet, and cybersex

Books, magazines, films, videos, music, advertisements, and internet images all can be aids to sexual excitement. They can make people feel happy, content in themselves, relaxed, focused, and stimulated whether they are alone or with a partner, but they can have many different meanings for those who use them. For example, a man who collects pornography may be unconsciously attacking his partner, whom he sees as not giving him everything that the models in the erotic imagery would.

The internet provides extremely easy access to many forms of sexual expression and sexual excitement to cater for all tastes, and "subscribers" never need leave their computer to explore these delights. For the sex addict, cybersex provides an Aladdin's cave of sexual activities. Some find that just looking at a computer or visiting a site that promises access to explicit material is sexually arousing. The internet offers a new freedom to explore sex and sexuality that can be positive and negative.

Chat rooms—Thousands of chat rooms are devoted to erotic sexual discussion or online pornography. Chat can be anonymous, explicit, and daring, with many ideas never likely to be discussed face to face.

Internet dating—Dating sites have personal details and photographs, and people can link up with their choice of partner, finding this an effective way of spending time with someone likeminded. This is quicker and perhaps more sophisticated than replying to box numbers or voicemails in newspapers or magazines.

The relationship is often back to front, however, in that people discuss many intimate details with each other over the internet before they meet in reality. Taboo subjects are easier to talk about with a stranger, but sex in the flesh may have to live up to that previously enjoyed on the net.

Therapists have noted an increasing addiction and compulsivity in cybersex. Some people spend many hours at work and at home surfing the net, masturbating to erotic

"The spanner case"

The police discovered a homemade video in which explicit gay sadomasochism performed by sadomasochistic participants was shown. After an investigation called "Operation Spanner," the participants were charged with "conspiracy to corrupt public morals" and then, more seriously, with Offences Against the Person Act. All the activities were carried out in private and were consensual. Nevertheless, Judge Rant ruled that consent was no defence to a charge of assault. Two appeals and, finally, the European Court of Human Rights upheld the verdict

Times 20 February 1997

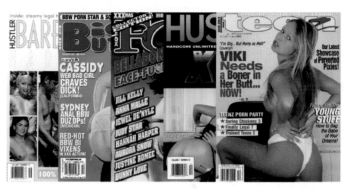
Magazines on the shelf

There is no established evidence to show that pornography makes people act out sociopathologically, such as causing men to commit rape

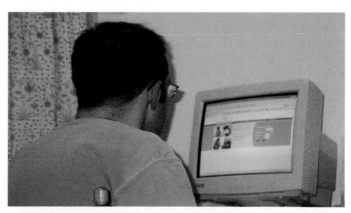
Internet dating is a fast and effective way of spending time with someone likeminded

imagery or while chatting to unknown people in chat rooms. Their partners may feel excluded, although the surfers feel they are not being unfaithful as this is "virtual" and not "real" sex.

Online dating agencies—Many such agencies exist and satisfy a need for shy and lonely people to meet other similar people. Dangers are obvious if they choose to meet, and people are advised to meet in a safe public place and not give any personal information until they feel secure with their chosen partner. Information given over the internet, of course, may not be true—witness the various recent cases of young people finding that their teenage date from the internet is in fact a considerably older person posing as a teenager.

Phone sex lines have to a degree been superceded by the much cheaper internet.

Paedophiles on the internet—this is the darker side of sex on the internet. Many people are aware of celebrities and unknown people alike who have been caught with downloaded pornographic images of children (downloading in this case means just having the images on the screen). Child pornography can be moving or still images, some that portray sex with young babies and others that show children being suspended in bondage equipment or penetrated by adults. As an inspector from the National Society for the Prevention of Cruelty to Children said "Behind these indecent, abusive images are real children who will have suffered immense damage and trauma."

Drugs used in sexual activity

The enjoyment of all the senses and the capacity of the human imagination lie at the basis of sexual stimulation, and some people will find simple massage with aromatic oils stimulating, while others will swear by special aphrodisiac foods such as oysters and shellfish. The use of drugs during sex is a large subject, but a focus on examples of clinical interest is useful.

Lidocaine is sold in sex shops as a spray to delay ejaculation. Its anaesthetic action, however, may well dull sensation in the partner who receives the penis.

Ecstasy (methylene dioxymethamphetamine)—Users report that their enjoyment of sex is heightened through an increase of loving feelings and that orgasm is delayed. A danger is that lowered inhibitions may lead to anal sex without the use of condoms and thus exposure to possible infection with HIV. Other amphetamines also produce euphoria, improve sexual functioning, and delay ejaculation.

Vasodilators (such as butyl nitrate, amyl nitrate, glyceryl trinitrate, and isosorbide dinitrate) in some forms are sold as "poppers" in small bottles (sometimes ampoules) from which vapour is inhaled. They work by liberation of nitrous oxide—a smooth muscle relaxant. A sensation of "rush" is experienced, which is followed by a short lived euphoria, with intensification of current positive emotions. They are often used by gay men, as muscle relaxation allows for easier anal intercourse and enhances orgasm. These drugs are suspected, but with no firm evidence, to depress the immune system. Concomitant use of sildenafil, vardenafil, or tadalafil is contraindicated totally because of a possibly lethal decrease in blood pressure.

Cocaine has been described as increasing sexual desire but making erection and ejaculation more difficult. If powder is placed on the glans or clitoris, cocaine acts as a local anaesthetic, delaying orgasm and prolonging intercourse. Placed within the anus, it has a similar anaesthetic effect, but the danger is that the receiver of a fist may be unaware of the pain and damage caused by too vigorous thrusting.

Cannabis is reported to enhance sexual feelings and the sense of touch, while increasing relaxation and pleasure.

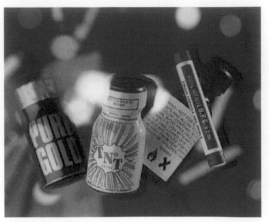

"Poppers" work by liberating nitrous oxide, which gives short lived euphoria with intensification of current positive emotions

---

Drugs used in sexual activity
- Lidocaine
- Ecstasy
- Vasodilators
- Cocaine
- Cannabis

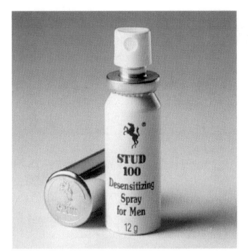

Sprays that incorporate lidocaine are used to delay ejaculation

A placebo effect seems to be present, with those who expect enhancement experiencing it, while those who have no such expectations do not.

The pictures of dildos, love balls, man in straightjacket, and breath control games are from the *Expectations* catalogue. The photograph of nipple, naval, pubic and scrotal piercings is reproduced from Ferguson H, *BMJ* 1999;319:1627-9. The photograph of a transvestite, by Anne Maniglier, is reproduced with permission of Gaze International. The photograph of the blindfolded man with ball gag and nipple clamps is courtesy of Housk Randall. The photographs of the inflatable doll and the tickler are courtesy of ABS Holdings catalogue. The cartoon of Wilbert is with permission of the Marie Stopes International. The internet dating photograph is courtesy of S Morgan.

18 Gender related disorders

Kevan Wylie

Some famous people are said to have had discomfort with their anatomical or assigned sex, including the Roman emperor Heliogabalus, James I of England, and Henry III of France. As long ago as Hippocrates' time in the 5th century BC, male to female gender changes were reported in a Caucasian tribe. Similar groups in ancient Tahitian tribes and American Indians were described as having special spiritual powers. The term gender dysphoria has been coined to describe this condition.

Herschvelt introduced the word transsexual in 1923, and the first sexual reassignment surgery was attempted in 1930. In 1954, Harry Benjamin noticed that many transsexual but non-psychotic men self castrated, and he championed the case for recognising the needs of transgendered people. He was the first psychiatrist to clearly distinguish transsexualism from homosexuality, although it remains a struggle for many transsexuals to gain awareness and acceptance. The description of transsexualism as a mental illness led eventually to the introduction of the term into the American Psychiatric Association's *Diagnostic and Statistical Manual of Mental Disorders*, third revision (DSM III), in 1980. Since then, the challenge has been to see whether this condition sits comfortably within the diagnosis of a mental disorder or as some other medical or endocrinological disorder.

Terminology

The designation of sex has always been established by looking at the anatomical sex and the term gender identity describes whether a person senses himself or herself to be either masculine or feminine. Gender role describes how people publicly express themselves in their clothing, use of cosmetics, hairstyle, conversation, body language, appearance, and behaviour. Usually, gender identity and gender role are congruous, but in people with gender identity disorder, severe incongruity exists between anatomical sex and gender identity, and the person has persistent discomfort with his or her anatomical sex, usually from childhood. A sense of inappropriateness is felt in the gender role of that sex, and such people have a strong, ongoing, crossgender identification, with a desire to live and be accepted as a member of the opposite sex. Usually they have a desire for hormonal therapy and surgery to make their body as congruent as possible with the desired gender identity.

It is essential to recognise that sexual orientation—the sex someone finds erotically attractive—is distinct from gender identity and role, and it may be heterosexual, homosexual, or bisexual. The proportion of heterosexual, bisexual, and gay people is no different in transgendered people than in non-transgendered people, and most studies suggest that heterosexuality occurs after surgical reassignment.[1]

Aetiology

The aetiology of gender dysphoria is controversial. Some believe the cause to reflect the physical and mental health of the mother during pregnancy, while others believe that a disturbed interaction occurs between parts of the brain and sex hormones during development of the foetus, as by the sixth week of gestation, brain sex is a reality, and gender programming may have started. Other theorists have described the condition to

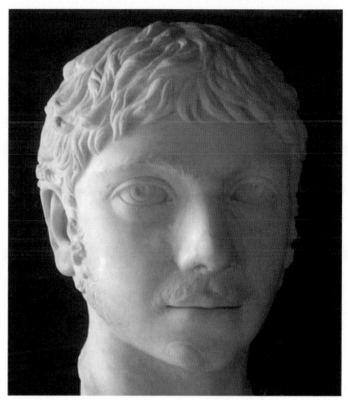

Heliogabalus—Roman emperor who was murdered by his own troops when he was 19 years old in 222 AD after a reign of four years of unparalleled debauchery

People who identify themselves with transsexualism are known as trans people. Those who are assigned as female at birth but who sense their body sexual function as, and identify themselves as, male are known as trans men, and vice versa. Once treatment through hormonal and surgical intervention is complete, many people no longer identify themselves as trans but simply as men or women

A delay in gender assignment with cosmetic surgery for intersex patients until the patient can give informed, adult consent is now generally accepted. In cases of doubt, such as intersexuality or hermaphrodism (in clinical cases, like adrenal hyperplasia or androgen resistance), however, determination of genetic sex is essential

reflect developmental problems during early life. There is an emphasis on the nurturing aspects of gender reinforcements and programming. Children may have to suppress their natural behaviours and tendencies to conform and fit in, which can cause undue distress.

Some evidence shows that transsexualism may be a neurodevelopmental condition during foetal growth. Several sexually dimorphic nuclei have been found in the hypothalamic area of the brain, particularly the sexually dimorphic limbic nucleus (the central subdivision of the bed nucleus of the stria terminalis) that becomes fully matured in the human brain by early adulthood.

One study found that the biological structure in the brains of male to female transsexual people had a totally female pattern that was not attributable to cross sex hormone therapy.[1] A second paper found that regardless of sexual orientation, men had almost twice as many somatostatin neurones as women.[2] These inhibit thyroid stimulating hormone and growth hormones in the hypothalamus, and the number of neurones in male to female transsexual people was similar to that in women, whereas the number of neurones in female to male transsexual people was similar to that in men. This seems to support a neurobiological basis for gender identity disorder.

Hormones may influence considerably the dimorphic development at several critical times: initially during the foetal period, around the time of birth, and, most likely, after birth. Contributors to an altered hormone environment may include genetic influences, medication, environmental influences, and stress of or trauma to the mother during pregnancy.

Where a predisposition for transsexualism exists, a variety of factors including psychosexual matters may subsequently play a role in outcome.

Regional variations

In South Asia, especially India and Bangladesh, *kothis*, although men, see themselves as feminine in a masculine-feminine sexual partnership, and they play out their perceived gender role as a female. By identifying as feminised males, *kothis* adapt social roles, mannerisms, and behaviour in ways that will attract what they call *panthis*—"real" men, who will sexually penetrate them but who will also have sex with women given the opportunity. The men who use *kothis* for sex, and sometimes for sexual relationships and partnerships, play the "dominant", "active," and "penetrating" roles. Sociocultural, religious, and family pressures ensure that most *kothis* eventually marry and produce children, no matter how long they attempt to delay this process. This intense pressure not surprisingly produces a range of major psychological effects.

In pre-modern Asian and Pacific Islander cultures, people who today would be identified as lesbian, gay, bisexual, transgender, or intersexual might have identified themselves as *bakla* (Tagalog), *shamakhami* (Bengali), *waria* (Javanese), *paksu mudang* (Korean), or *mahu* (Hawaiian). European colonialism had a deleterious effect on many traditions of transgender in Asia and the Pacific. The Babain culture of transgendered priests and priestesses revered in traditional Filipino society was destroyed by Catholic missionaries in the nineteenth century and the mahus (usually one per village) have disappeared or, as in Tahiti, lost their honoured position in society.

Differential diagnosis

Tranvestism

In cross-dressing transvestism, men find intense relief in dressing in women's clothing. In these circumstances,

> When a predisposition for transsexualism exists, a variety of factors, including psychosocial factors, may play a role in outcome

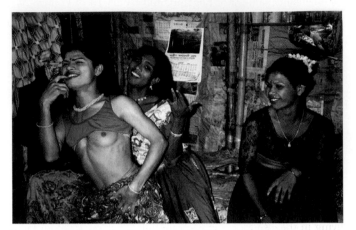

These are not transvestites or transsexuals. They are *Sylhet kothis*, who although men, see themselves as feminine and adopt mannerisms to attract *panthis*—real men. With permission of Naz Foundation International

> Being a *panthi* says more about sexual practices than sexual identity. Many are married men or are men who are heterosexually active but unmarried and occasionally prefer sex with a younger man. In a culture that socially protects women, excluding them from public spaces and controlling male access to them, sexual gratification for many "manly" males has to be with *kothis*, or those deemed less "manly"—young men and adolescents. They do not see themselves as homosexual or less masculine, because the people they have sex with are not men, but feminised males—they are *kothis*, who are not "real" men. The sex or gender identity of paid partners seems to be irrelevant as long as they are available for rapid and cheap penetrative sex, but this produces a worrying amount of sexually transmitted disease, especially HIV, and local trauma

Case example of transvestite fetishism from Krafft-Ebing (1887)

J, a young butcher, when arrested, was found to be wearing underneath his overcoat a bodice, a corset, a vest, a jacket, a collar, a jersey and a chemise, also fine stockings and garters. Since he was eleven, he was troubled by the desire to wear a chemise of his elder sister. Whenever he could do it unnoticed, he indulged in this pleasure, and since the age of puberty, the wearing of such a garment would bring on ejaculation. When he became independent, he bought chemises and other articles of female toilet. To put on such garments was the great aim of his sexual instinct and he begged the hospital physician to let him wear female attire.

progression to sexual arousal and activity or an intense desire to seek sexual reassignment surgery is rare. In transvestite fetishism, the person, who is almost invariably a man, obtains sexual arousal as a consequence of dressing in women's clothing. Masturbation or other sexual activity associated with the crossdressing is not unusual, with the man later discarding the clothing, often with a degree of repulsion.

Legal issues

In the United Kingdom in 1970, a legal judgement removed the right to correct birth certificates. This meant that trans people lost their rights to marry, foster, adopt, and receive support from domestic violence. Custodial sentencing placements also were affected.

In 1998, a legal judgement from the European Court of Justice meant that discrimination on grounds of a person's transsexualism became illegal, and rights were put in effect by the Sex Discrimination (Gender Reassignment) Regulations that year.

The Gender Recognition Act 2004 makes provision for a person of either gender, aged at least 18, to make an application for a gender recognition certificate on the basis of living in the gender other than identified on the original birth certificate. A diagnosis of gender dysphoria and evidence of having lived in the acquired gender for at least two years will be necessary. It will not be necessary for full gender reassignment surgery to have taken place. A short certificate of birth can then be issued.

Standards of care

The Harry Benjamin International Gender Dysphoria Association laid out internationally agreed standards of care for transgendered patients who want to change to their chosen gender.[3] These standards outline the pathways of treatment that should be available to patients seeking help in the transition. They include the role of the mental health professional to diagnose accurately any comorbid psychiatric conditions, confirm the gender disorder, and ensure that patients are offered appropriate treatment. Evidence shows that one in ten trans people may have problems with mental illness, genital mutilation, or suicide attempts. Trans people should be counselled about the range of treatment options and implications and, where necessary, should be encouraged to have psychotherapy. The professional should ascertain eligibility and readiness for progression to hormone and surgical therapy. Wherever possible, this should be done within the context of a multidisciplinary team and should take into account individual patient needs rather than enforcing a rigid package of care.

Patients are deemed ready to receive hormone therapy when they have fulfilled three conditions.

- They have had the opportunity of further consolidation of their chosen gender identity with psychotherapy or real life experience in the preferred gender role
- They have made progress in mastering other identified problems that lead to improvements in or continuing stable mental health
- They are likely to take hormones in a responsible manner.

The real life experience can happen at a predetermined time or before starting hormonal therapy; the decision usually depends on local policy. The person must aim to maintain

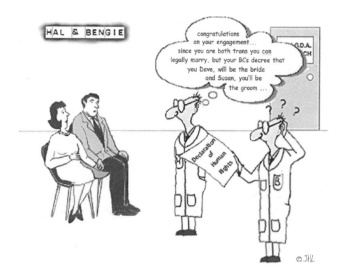

Drugs often used in gender clinics

Masculinisation
- Testosterone 250 mg intramuscularly every three weeks or transdermal patches or gels

Feminisation
Aged < 40 years
- Estradiol 0.5-2 mg once to three times daily to establish satisfactory serum levels

Aged ≥ 40 years
- Estradiol transdermal system 25-100 mcg patch (Estraderm TTX) applied to the skin and changed twice weekly

In addition, for all age groups, an antiandrogen, such as cyproterone acetate 50 mg 1-2 tablets daily or spironolactone 100 mg once daily, may be necessary

Patients must be fully counselled about the off licence status of these drugs

---

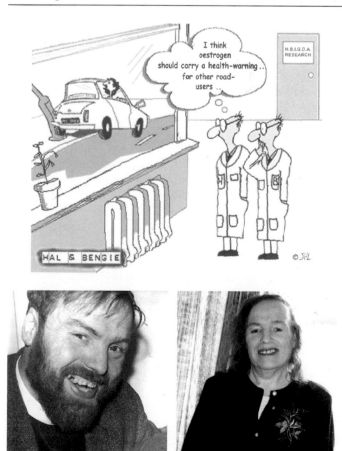

Reverend WD Parry. Trans female (before and after sex change)

full-time or part-time employment or function as a student or in a community based volunteer activity.

He or she must provide written documentation to prove that people other than the therapists acknowledge that the patient successfully passes and functions in the chosen gender role. Those who are retired may have some problems in providing such documentation.

Clear guidelines about haematological, biochemical, and endocrinological monitoring should be given before and during treatment with hormones.[4] When starting hormonal therapy, the desired effects and the positive and negative side effects must be outlined to the patient and appropriate consent should be obtained. It is good practice to ensure that any partner of the patient is aware of the effects of prescribed medications. Reproductive options with gamete storage should be taken into account and explicit consent obtained. Speech and language therapy and hair removal techniques should be offered at this stage.

Gender reassignment surgery

After a minimum of 12 months' supervision within the real life experience, the opportunity for surgery can be considered. As with entering hormonal therapy, criteria of eligibility and readiness need to be met. When the supervising team is convinced that these have been satisfied, a second psychiatric or medical opinion should be sought, preferably from an experienced clinician from another service. If this opinion is supportive, the patients should be referred to a specialist surgeon. Surgical options include breast surgery and genital reassignment surgery. The patient must be fully counselled about the limitations of surgery and the potential complications.

Trans men may be offered bilateral mastectomy, hysterectomy, oöphorectomy, and fashioning a new penis and scrotum. Possible operations for trans women are removal of the penis and testes and fashioning a new vagina and clitoris, as well as techniques such as breast augmentation, reshaping of the nose and the cricothyroid cartilages, facial remodelling, and hair transplants. Adequate post-operative care from the surgical, hormonal, and therapeutic points of view must be provided.

Studies that have reported the outcome of sex reassignment surgery have found varied results. One report suggests satisfaction with the surgical results in 87% of male to female patients and 97% of female to male patients, although different studies report different results. Young age, good family and social support, and success of the surgical procedures are all factors that correlate with patients' long term satisfaction.[5]

Summary

Gender identity disorder is a condition being given greater attention and importance by the medical profession. Although its aetiology is unclear, some evidence suggests that it has a neurobiological basis. The condition is no longer confused with sexual orientation preference and other gender related disorders. Although social stigmata remain, recognition of the need for multidisciplinary teams in the assessment and care of patients throughout their real life experience is apparent.

1 Zhou J-N, Hofman MA, Gooren LJG, Swaab DF. A sex difference in the human brain and its relation to transsexuality. *Nature* 1995;378:68-70
2 Kruijver FPM, Zhou J-N, Pool CW, Hofman MA, Gooren LJG, Swaab DF. Male to female transsexuals have female neuron numbers in a limbic nucleus. *J Clin Endocrinol Metab* 2000;85: 2034-41

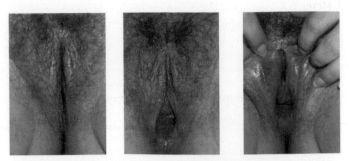

Male to female surgery. With permission of David Ralph

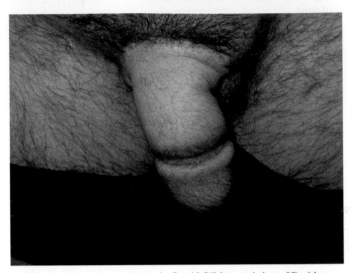

Female to male surgery—new penis: flaccid. With permission of David Ralph

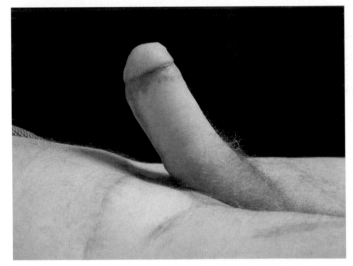

Female to male surgery—new penis: erect. With permission of David Ralph

Further reading

- Blanchard R, Steiner BW. *Clinical management of gender identity disorders in children and adults.* Washington: American Psychiatric Press, 1990. www.symposion.com/ijt/soc_2001/index.htm
- Blanchard R, Federoff JP. The case for and against publicly funded transsexual surgery. *Psych Rounds* 2000;4:2
- Nanda S. *Neither man nor woman—Hijiras of India.* New York: Wadsworth Publishing, 1990
- Jaffrey Z. *The invisibles—a tale of the eunuchs of India.* London: Weidenfeld, and Nicholson, 1997
- Department for Constitutional Affairs. *Government policy concerning transsexual people.* London: Department for Constitutional Affairs, 2004. http://www.dca.gov.uk/constitution/transsex/policy.htm

3 Meyer W III, Bockting WO, Cohen-Kettenis P, Coleman E. The standards of care for gender identity disorders (sixth version). *Int J Transgenderism* 2001;5:1

4 Ceglie D, Devor H, et al. The standards of care for gender identity disorders (sixth version). *Int J Transgenderism* 2001;5:1

5 Futterweit W. Endocrine therapy of transsexuals and potential complications of long term treatment. *Arch Sex Behaviour* 1998;27:209-26

Hal & Bengie cartoons courtesy of Dr Jay Hayes-Light, Director of UKIA

Support networks

A variety of support networks exist for patients undergoing gender transition.

- The Gender Trust offers information and support to transsexual, gender dysphoric, and transgender people. The trust is a registered charity established in 1990 and is unique in the areas of work it covers (http://www.gendertrust.org.uk/)
- The FTM Network is an informal and ad hoc self help group, open to all female to male transgender and transsexual people, or those exploring this aspect of their gender (email: s.t.whittle@mmu.ac.uk)
- The Beaumont Society was founded in 1966 and is the world's largest membership organisation for crossdressers, transvestites, and transsexuals. Support is also offered for wives and partners (http://www.beaumontsociety.org.uk/)
- Mermaids is a support group for gender variant children and teenagers. Their aim is to support children and teenagers up to the age of 19 who are trying to cope with gender identity issues. They also offer support to parents, families, carers, and others (http://www.mermaids.freuk.com)
- CHANGE is a support group run by volunteers. Its aim is to improve the quality of life for those with transsexual syndrome (http://members.aol.com/ts1change/homepage.htm
- GIRES (Gender Identity Research and Education Society) offers support to all family members with a close relative with gender identity disorders (http://www.gires.org.uk)
- Press for Change is a political lobbying and educational organisation, which campaigns to achieve equal civil rights and liberties for all transgender people in the United Kingdom, through legislation and social change (http://www.pfc.org.uk/)
- Naz Foundation International is an organisation set up to help *kothis* physically and medically (http://www.nfi.net)

19 Hormone replacement in women and men

Margaret Rees, John M Tomlinson

Hormone replacement in women

Menopause and its consequences

Menopause is the permanent cessation of menstruation that results from loss of ovarian follicular activity; the median age at which it occurs is 51 years. Increasing life expectancy means that women can expect more than 30 years of post-menopausal life.[1]

Decline in concentrations of oestrogen at the menopause can cause acute menopausal symptoms. About 70% of women in western cultures will experience vasomotor symptoms, such as hot flushes and night sweats. Other symptoms include tiredness, depressed mood, loss of libido, and lethargy. The long term complications of the menopause, such as osteoporosis, may have a greater bearing on a woman's quality and even quantity of life than the acute short term symptoms.

What is hormone replacement therapy?

Hormone replacement therapy (HRT) consists of an oestrogen that in non-hysterectomised women is combined with a progestogen. This is added to the oestrogen to reduce the increased risk of endometrial hyperplasia and carcinoma that occurs with unopposed oestrogen, and so it does not need to be given to hysterectomised women.[1,2] HRT is given cyclically, which causes a menstrual like bleed, or continuously, with the oestrogen causing amenorrhoea. Addition of progestogen can be for 10-14 days every four weeks, 14 days every 13 weeks, or every day continuously. Different routes of administration are used: oral, transdermal, subcutaneous, intranasal, and vaginal.

Low dose natural oestrogens, such as vaginal oestriol creams or pessaries or oestradiol by tablet or ring, can be used to treat urogenital symptoms. No adverse endometrial effects should occur with recommended dose regimens, and a progestogen need not be added for endometrial protection. Tibolone is a synthetic steroid with mixed oestrogenic, progestogenic, and androgenic actions that is used in postmenopausal women who wish to have amenorrhoea. It is used to treat vasomotor symptoms, psychological problems, and sexual drive problems.

Hormone replacement therapy is a controversial area because of publications from the randomised Women's Health Initiative in 2002 and the observational Million Women Study in 2003.[3-5] Women's Health Initiative was designed in the early 1990s to work out ways of preventing and controlling some of the most common causes of morbidity and mortality among healthy postmenopausal women aged 50-79 years. It also considered calcium and vitamin D supplementation and diets with low fat content, as well as hormone replacement therapy. It is only the oestrogen and progestogen part of the trial that was stopped after five years, because the risk of invasive breast cancer exceeded the predetermined safety threshold, but the lack of benefit in prevention of cardiovascular disease, previously found in other observational studies, has attracted the most attention. The other parts of the trial, including oestrogen alone, continue. The Million Women Study obtained information from women aged 50-64 years who attended the NHS Breast Screening Programme in the United Kingdom.

The publicity that surrounds these studies makes it essential to assess them critically and not generically extrapolate the results of a single study to all menopausal women.

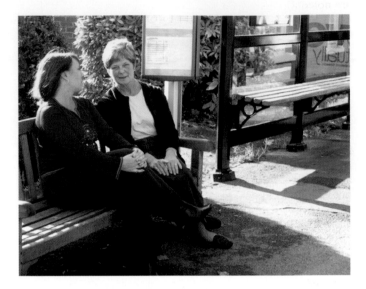

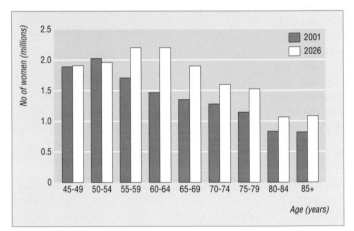

Increase in women aged over 45 years predicted to occur in United Kingdom by 2026. Adapted from Office for National Statistics and Government Actuaries Department 2002

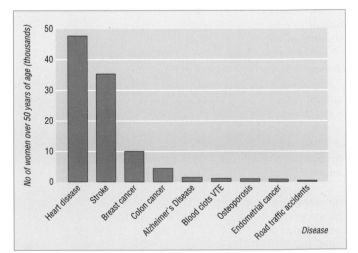

Main causes of death in women over 50 years of age in England and Wales in 2000. Numbers for Alzheimer's disease and osteoporosis are probably underestimated because they are often not accurately reported on death certificates. Office for National Statistics. Mortality statistics cause: review of the Registrar General on deaths by cause, sex and age, in England and Wales, 2000:Series DH2 no. 27

Benefits of HRT

HRT improves menopausal symptoms, prevents osteoporotic fractures, and reduces bowel cancer risk. Good evidence from randomised, placebo controlled studies shows that oestrogen is effective in dealing with hot flushes and improvements usually are noted within four weeks.[5] Hot flushes are the most common indication for HRT, and oestrogen often can be used for fewer than five years.

Randomised controlled trials (including the Women's Health Initiative) showed that oestrogen reduces the risk of spine, hip, and other fractures related to osteoporosis.[3,5] The most recent studies suggest that HRT must be given continuously and for life to prevent fractures effectively.[5] Although alternatives to HRT exist to prevent and treat osteoporosis, oestrogen may remain the best option particularly in young women or symptomatic women, or both. Hormone replacement therapy reduces the risk of colorectal cancer by about one third.[3] Sexuality may improve with oestrogen alone but may need addition of testosterone.

Risks of HRT

HRT and breast cancer

The risk of a woman developing breast cancer is considerably higher with current use of any type of HRT when the treatment is started in women aged >50 years and is similar to that associated with a late natural menopause. Such an effect is not seen in women who start hormone replacement therapy early for premature menopause; this indicates that duration of lifetime oestrogen exposure is relevant.

Addition of progestogen increases the risk of *breast* cancer over that with oestrogen alone. This must be balanced against the reduced risk of *endometrial* cancer with combined therapy. The risk of breast cancer falls after HRT is stopped; after five years, the risk is no greater than in women who do not take it.

In contrast with the Women's Health Initiative, the Million Women Study found a higher risk of breast cancer with all types of hormone replacement therapy (unopposed oestrogen, combined, and tibolone). The greatest risk was in women who took combined HRT. The Million Women Study's estimates of higher risk compared with the randomised Women's Health Initiative study probably reflect the observational nature of the former, and findings could be biased if differences existed between participants and non-participants. Randomised controlled trials are unlikely ever to be big enough to estimate reliably the effect of hormone replacement therapy on mortality, but observational studies do not show an adverse outcome on survival.

Hormone replacement therapy and endometrial cancer

Unopposed oestrogen replacement increases the risk of endometrial cancer. The risk is not completely eliminated with monthly sequential addition of progestogen, especially when used for more than five years. This also was found with long cycle HRT (with progestogen every three months). Continuous combined regimens showed no increased risk of endometrial cancer.

Hormone replacement therapy and venous thromboembolism

Hormone replacement therapy increases the risk of venous thromboembolism (deep vein thrombosis and pulmonary embolism) by twofold. The highest risk occurs in the first year of use. Women who have previously had venous thromboembolism have an increased risk of recurrence, especially in the first year of use.

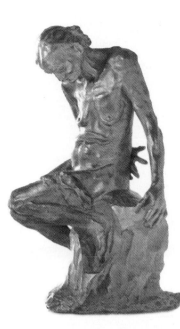

Celle qui fut la belle heaulmière.
Bronze by Auguste Rodin, 1885.
Photograph by Henri Martinie
(1897-1965)

Symptoms that respond well to topical or systemic oestrogens

- Vaginal dryness
- Soreness
- Superficial dyspareunia
- Urinary frequency
- Urinary urgency

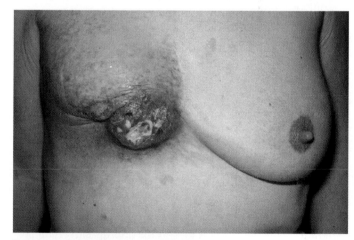

Carcinoma of right breast

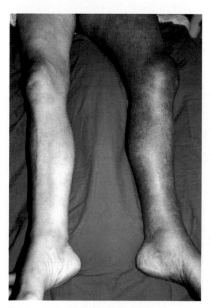

Deep vein thrombosis

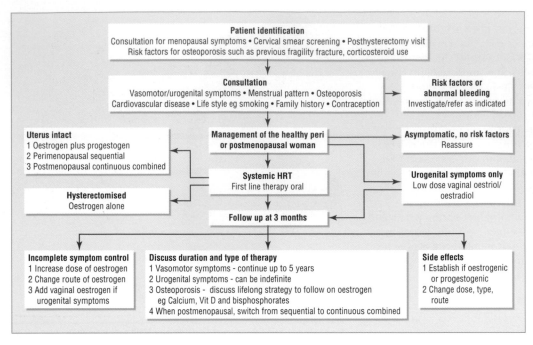

Management and treatment of the peri- and postmenopausal woman

Uncertainties about HRT

Previously thought to be protective, the role of hormone replacement therapy in coronary heart disease and stroke in primary or secondary prevention has now become uncertain so it should not be used primarily for these indications.[3,6]

Several studies suggested that use of oestrogen may delay or prevent onset of Alzheimer's disease.[7] In contrast, the Women's Health Initiative found a twofold increased risk of dementia in women who took combined therapy.[3] This increased risk was only significant, however, in the group of women aged >75 years. This contradiction with previous studies may be because a critical time for an effect of oestrogen exists in the disease process.

Most data about ovarian cancer relate to replacement with oestrogen alone, with increasing risk in the very long term (>10 years). With continuous combined therapy, however, this increase does not seem so apparent.[5]

Conclusion

Hormone replacement therapy still offers the potential for benefit to outweigh harm as long as the appropriate regimen is instigated in terms of dose, route, and combination. Women with early ovarian failure should normally be offered HRT until the average age of menopause, at which point the treatment should be reassessed. The woman then needs to decide whether to stop or continue the treatment.

Testosterone replacement in men

Testosterone replacement in men is causing a lot of debate; it is not helped by the use of terms such as the "midlife crisis", the "male menopause," and the "andropause" and the fact that the media have decided that the use of testosterone supplements will keep a man looking and feeling younger, help his sex life, and cure his impotence.

What are the facts?

It is important to define the terms. The midlife crisis is a psychological state that occurs in some men who, having reached their forties, feel that life is slipping away without much achievement and with goals unattained and dreams unachieved. The male menopause and the andropause are inaccurate terms.

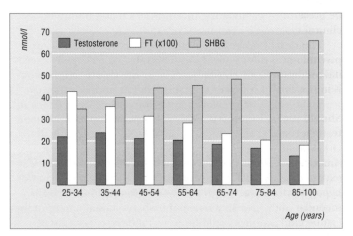

Mean serum levels of testosterone, free testosterone (FT) and sex hormone binding globulin (SHBG) according to age in a cross sectional study of 300 healthy men. Adapted from Verumeula A et al. *J Clin Endocrinol Metab* 1996;81:1821-7

Comparison of menopause and andropause

Menopause	Andropause
• Reduced sex drive and enjoyment	• Reduced sex drive with a marked decrease in erectile quality, especially nocturnal and early morning erections
• Mental and physical fatigue	• Tiredness, exhaustion, loss of concentration, decrease in intellectual ability
• Mood swings	• Irritability and anger
• Depression (sometimes severe)	• Depression (sometimes severe)
• Aches and pains	• Muscle aches and joint pains
• Hot flushes	• Hot flushes and red face
• Severe sweating, especially at night	• Severe sweating, especially at night

There is no "pause" in men as in a woman's climacteric. No rapid diminution of hormone production occurs over a short period as in women (except occasionally because of major trauma). More appropriate terms, "partial androgen deficiency in the adult male" or "post-pubertal hypogonadism" are clumsy, however, so the term andropause seems to have caught on. To accept that there is such an entity as the andropause (and many hotly deny its existence), it must be defined carefully.

Production of testosterone is governed by the hypothalamus through the pituitary, with the production of a chemical messenger, luteinising hormone, which acts on Leydig cells in the testes. This is a self governing, reciprocal action, so that if testosterone falls below a certain level, luteinising hormone increases to stimulate further production of testosterone. It is now accepted that a man's testosterone level tends to diminish slowly, with the mean serum concentrations at age 75 years being about two thirds of those at age 25 years. Nevertheless great variability is seen, with some fit elderly men having serum concentrations of testosterone well within the normal range for young adults.

What does partial androgen deficiency entail? Symptoms in some men closely parallel menopausal symptoms in women with oestrogen deficiency. Other more nebulous features are a decrease of energy and virility, marked loss of drive (general or sexual), loss of sexual fantasies, loss of muscle bulk and strength, an increase in upper and central body fat, and a feeling of being "out of sorts." Not all of these symptoms may be present, and some may be more severe than others, so a clinical diagnosis should be supported by biochemical tests.

The causes are manifold and include physiological and psychological causes, as well as increasing age. Which men will have symptoms severe enough to ask for help, and at what age, is impossible to predict.

Should men with secondary low concentrations of testosterone be treated?

Great polarisation of opinion exists on who to treat. One American endocrinologist said the andropause is "a myth to excuse the lazy and unfit."[8] Some doctors feel that only primary hypogonadism (such as Kleinfelter's syndrome) and severe secondary hypogonadism should be treated, as the symptoms can be explained on other grounds. Others believe that men of any age with these symptoms and low concentrations of testosterone suffer severely—mentally and physically—with a loss of work output and a fall in quality of life and effectiveness in society that can be reversed by testosterone supplementation.[9] Replacement in the past has been given to help impotence. When this did not succeed or caused side effects, it fell out of favour and gained a tarnished reputation. Replacement has therefore to be justified, instigated, and monitored carefully.

Justification for treatment

Justification for treatment is sometimes difficult and it depends on taking a careful history, doing a thorough examination (including rectal examination of the prostate), and blood tests, which should also include the concentration of testosterone, sex hormone binding globulin, and the free androgen index. As levels of sex hormone binding globulin increase with age, free testosterone levels fall. Guidelines of the International Society for the Ageing Male suggest that replacement testosterone should be given if the serum concentrations of testosterone fall much below 11 nmol/l.[10]

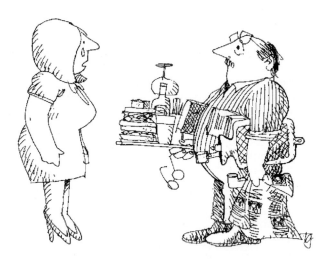

"I REMEMBER WHEN, THE ONLY THING YOU WANTED TO TAKE TO BED, WAS ME!"

Some secondary causes of low testosterone

Physiological	Psychological
• Diabetes and obesity	• Bereavement
• Alcohol misuse	• Divorce
• Infections (mumps, sexually transmitted diseases, and HIV and AIDS)	• Loss of employment
• Physical trauma (road traffic accidents) and major operations	• Acute family stresses
• Myocardial infarction	

Advantages and disadvantages of preparations

Preparations	Advantages	Disadvantages
Capsules	Easy to take (40 mg testosterone undecanoate three times daily with food) Rapid onset	Need to be taken three times daily with food Supraphysiological and subphysiological swings of testosterone within hours are unpleasant
Injections	Only once every two-three weeks (testosterone enanthate 250 mg or testosterone propionate mixtures) New three monthly injection to be launched soon	Similar swings at longer intervals Can be inconvenient for active people Needs a minor operation
Implants	600-1200 mg but compressed only once every 5-6 months Crystalline testosterone (100-200 mg)	Same swings as above
Patches	Easy to put on (2.5-5 mg/patch) Changed daily Rapid, even absorption of testosterone	Crackles with movement 50% have a reaction to patch (not to testosterone)
Transdermal gel	Easy to put on, 50 mg/ 5 ml rubbed in daily No swings	Occasionally sensitivity to gel
Sachet	Rapid, even absorption and improvement of symptoms	

Instigation of treatment

A range of testosterone preparations (capsules, injections, patches, implants, and now transdermal preparations) is available.

Monitoring of treatment

There is widespread anxiety that giving testosterone may cause carcinoma of the prostate. So far this never has been proved,[11] but, as carcinoma of the prostate is androgen dependent, pre-existing prostate carcinoma can be aggravated. A pretreatment measurement of prostate specific antigen (PSA) is therefore essential, and this should be followed by a repeat measurement if the first is raised (no matter how slight the original increase). It should be repeated after three months and then annually. This is an unsatisfactory test, however, as only 30% of patients with raised levels have a carcinoma. The concentrations also can be raised for 72 hours after ejaculation and in patients with sexually transmitted infections, benign hypertrophy, or in long distance cyclists.

Testosterone misuse

Doctors and allied professionals need to be aware that misuse of anabolic androgenic steroids and pituitary hormones by sports people is widespread (although it is hotly denied in public), with participants in bodybuilding, athletics, cycling, rugby, and association football among the misusers.[12] Such misuse is most noticeable in competitive bodybuilding, with the incidence of use estimated at 25-50% (although this may be an underestimate), as the aim is to impress competition judges and peers. The drugs are easily accessible, with most brought into the United Kingdom from Greece, Mexico, and Brazil, where they can be bought over the counter without prescription, and sold on the black market here.

Very large doses are used. Throughout a year, a keen bodybuilder may inject up to 10 ampoules of testosterone proprionate a week (normal therapeutic dose is three ampoules per week) and 4-6 ampoules of a 250 mg mixture of testosterone esters weekly (Sustanon 100 or 250) (normal dose is one every three weeks) with the addition of 20 tablets of stanozolol (Stromba) 5 mg daily (normal dose is two tablets daily) and mesterolone (Pro-Viron) 250 mg daily (normal dose is 75 mg daily) before a show to "sculpt" the muscles. In addition, if he can afford it, he will use growth hormone 2 mg a day (equivalent to 6 IU) at a daily cost of about £25 to "burn" fat and build muscles. (For athletes who take growth hormone illicitly, it has the advantage that currently it is difficult to detect. Randomised controlled trials have shown, however, that muscle strength and size are no better than could be achieved with strenuous exercise in fit young men.[12])

Men who take long term steroids and worry about shrinking testes stop every three months and take human chorionic gonadotrophin, 1500 units three times a week for one week. Stopping the steroids allows natural recovery, but this can take months. Diuretics and ephedrine also are taken to try to minimise fluid retention, and tamoxifen 20 mg daily is used to avoid gynaecomastia ("bitch tits"). The prizes for winning a major bodybuilding contest are great—£30 000 in the United Kingdom and £200 000 for a world title.

The physical dangers are great. Most bodybuilders know someone who has had cardiovascular symptoms such as cardiomyopathy at an early age or died young from myocardial infarction, and former East German athletes had their lives severely damaged by state sponsored drugging. Shrinking of testes and sterility are also common side effects of continued excessive male hormone dosage. If taken in adolescence they can cause premature epiphyseal closure and permanent stunting in height. Long term overdosage can also lead to a rise

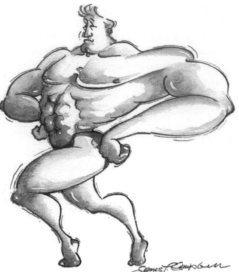

Muscle strength and size are no better than could be achieved by strenuous exercise in healthy young men

For top players in all major sports, the financial rewards are great. For a player of such sports to feel he cannot be as good as the others unless he too succumbs is very tempting, and many do succumb, but random testing now is more frequent and thorough. Many recent designer drugs, such as sublingual tetrahydrogestrinone (generally known as THG), however, have been detected only recently as more sophisticated tests have been developed

Side effects of steroid misuse

Men	Women
• Cardiovascular symptoms (cardiomyopathy and myocardial infarction)	• Menstrual problems • Virilisation
• Shrinking of testes	• Irreversible hirsutism
• Sterility	• Male pattern baldness
• Premature epiphyseal closure and permanent stunting of height when taken during adolescence	• Deepening voice • Enlarged clitoris
• Rises in haematocrit, with possible embolism, liver damage, and severe troublesome cystic acne with scarring	

in heamatocrit with possible embolism, liver damage and severe troublesome cystic acne with scarring.

Women also can suffer problems from testosterone misuse. Those who take male hormones to excess can suffer from menstrual problems as well as virilisation with irreversible hirsutism, male pattern baldness, deepening voice and an enlarged clitoris.

Conclusion

A large number of men who need testosterone replacement do not get it, largely because the problem is not recognised or many doctors feel that to treat an older man with testosterone wastes money on a lifestyle problem. There is no proof that testosterone in appropriate doses shortens life and to prevent a hypogonadal patient from receiving the necessary substitution would force him to continue a miserable life of low quality.[9] Those who are treated, however, are grateful (as are their families) for the vast improvement in their general well being. There is no medical justification for withholding the benefits of substitutive treatment from symptomatic hypogonadal elderly men.[13]

1 Rees M, Purdie DW. *Management of the menopause*. Marlow: British Menopause Society Publications, 2002

2 Weiderpass E, Adami HO, Baron JA, Magnusson C, Bergstrom R, Lindgren A, et al. Risk of endometrial cancer following estrogen replacement with and without progestins. *J Natl Cancer Inst* 1999;91:1131-7

3 Writing Group for the Women's Health Initiative Investigators. Risks and benefits of estrogen plus progestin in healthy postmenopausal women: principal results from the Women's Health Initiative randomized controlled trial. *JAMA* 2002; 288:321-33

4 Million Women Study Collaborators. Breast cancer and hormone-replacement therapy in the Million Women Study. *Lancet* 2003;362:419-27

5 Managing the menopause: British Menopause Society Council consensus statement on hormone replacement therapy. *J Br Menopause Soc* 2003;9:129-31

6 Mosca L, Collins P, Herrington DM, Mendelsohn ME, Pasternak RC, Robertson RM, et al. Hormone replacement therapy and cardiovascular disease: a statement for healthcare professionals from the American Heart Association. *Circulation* 2001; 104:499-503

7 Kesslak JP. Can estrogen play a significant role in the prevention of Alzheimer's disease? *J Neural Transm Suppl* 2002;62:227-39

8 Marsh B. "Menopause in men: a myth to excuse the lazy and unfit." quoting Prof J. McKinlay, *Daily Mail* 2003 p19, 17 July

9 Kaufman JM, Vermeulen A. Androgens in male senescence. In: Nieschlag E, Behre HM, eds. *Testosterone—action, deficiency, substitution*. Berlin and London: Springer, 1999:305

10 Cuzin B, Giuliano F, Jamin Ch, Legros JJ, Lejeune H, Rigot JM, et al. Investigation, treatment and monitoring of late-onset hypogonadism in males: the official guidelines of the International Society for the Study of the Aging Male (ISSAM) with comments. *Ann Endocrinol (Paris)* 2003;64:289-304

11 Slater S, Oliver RT. Testosterone: its role in development of prostate cancer and potential risk from use as hormone replacement therapy. *Drugs Ageing* 2000;17:431-9

12 Korkia P, Stimson GV. Indications of prevalence, practice and effects of anabolic steroid use in Great Britain. *Int J Sports Med* 1997;18:557-62

13 Kaufman JM, T'Sjoen G, Vermeulen A. Androgens in male senescence. In: Nieschlag E, Behre HM, eds. *Testosterone—action, deficiency, substitution*. Cambridge: Cambridge University Press, 2004: 518

Recommended reading and useful websites for health workers

- Rees M, Purdie DW. *Management of the menopause*. Marlow: British Menopause Society Publications, 2002

- Rees M, Purdie DW. *Management of the menopause. An integrated healthcare pathway for the management of the menopausal woman in primary care*. Marlow: British Menopause Society Publications, 2002. This excellent four page set of guidelines and summary of the management of the menopause is available from British Menopause Society, 4-6 Eton Place, Marlow, Bucks Sl7 2QA (www.the-bms.org.uk)

- Nieschlag E, Behre HM, eds. *Testosterone, action, deficiency, substitution*. Cambridge: Cambridge University Press, 2004. A very practical, thorough review of all aspects of testosterone

- Medical aspects of drug use in the gym. *Drug Ther Bull* 2004;42: 1-5. An excellent summary of all performance enhancing drugs used by athletes and bodybuilders

- A list of substances allowed and banned in competitive sports is available from UK Sport, 40 Bernard Street, London WC1N 1ST (www.uksport.gov.uk)

- British Menopause Society, 4-6 Eton Place, Marlow, Bucks Sl7 2QA (www.the-bms.org.uk)

- Men's Health Forum, Tavistock House, Tavistock Square, London WC1H 9HR (tel: 020 7388 4449; www. menshealthforum. org.uk). A comprehensive site for all male heath problems for health professionals and patients

- Sexual Dysfunction Association (formerly Impotence Association) (helpline: 0870 774 3571; theia@btinternet.com; www.impotence.org.uk). Deals with male and female sexual problems, with a telephone hotline for doctors and patients

- Institute of Psychosexual Medicine, 12 Chandos Street, London W1G 9DR (tel: 020 7580 0631; www.ipm.org.uk). Provides psychosexual training throughout the UK for doctors

- British Association of Sexual and Relationship Therapists, PO Box 13686, London, SW20 9ZH (www.basrt.org.uk). Promotes the education and training of clinicians and therapists who work in the fields of sexual and couple relationships, sexual dysfunction, and sexual health

Recommended reading and useful websites for patients and their partners

- Rees M, Purdie DW, Hope S. *The menopause—what you need to know*. Marlow: BMS Publications on behalf of The British Menopause Society, 2003. A small, very readable, and informative booklet for interested patients and their partners

- Women's Health Concern, PO Box 2126, Marlow SL7 2RY0 (helpline: 01628 483612; www. womens-health-concern.org.uk). Gives an up to date and authoritative view on women's health

- Men's Health Forum, Tavistock House, Tavistock Square, London WC1H 9HR (tel: 020 7388 4449; www. menshealthforum.org.uk). A comprehensive site for all male heath problems for health professionals and patients

- Sexual Dysfunction Association (formerly Impotence Association). Deals with male and female sexual problems, with a telephone hotline for doctors and patients (helpline: 0870 774 3571; theia@btinternet.com; www.impotence.org.uk

The cartoon 'I can remember when .....' is with permission of Tony Goffe. The cartoon of the body builder is with permission of Christina Bishop and James Campbell of the *Men's Health Journal*. The photograph of a carcinoma of the right breast is with permission of Mr Dick Rainsford

Index

Notes: As sexual health is the subject of this book, all index entries refer to this unless otherwise indicated. Page references in *italics* refer to figures, tables or boxed material.

Index

Index

Index